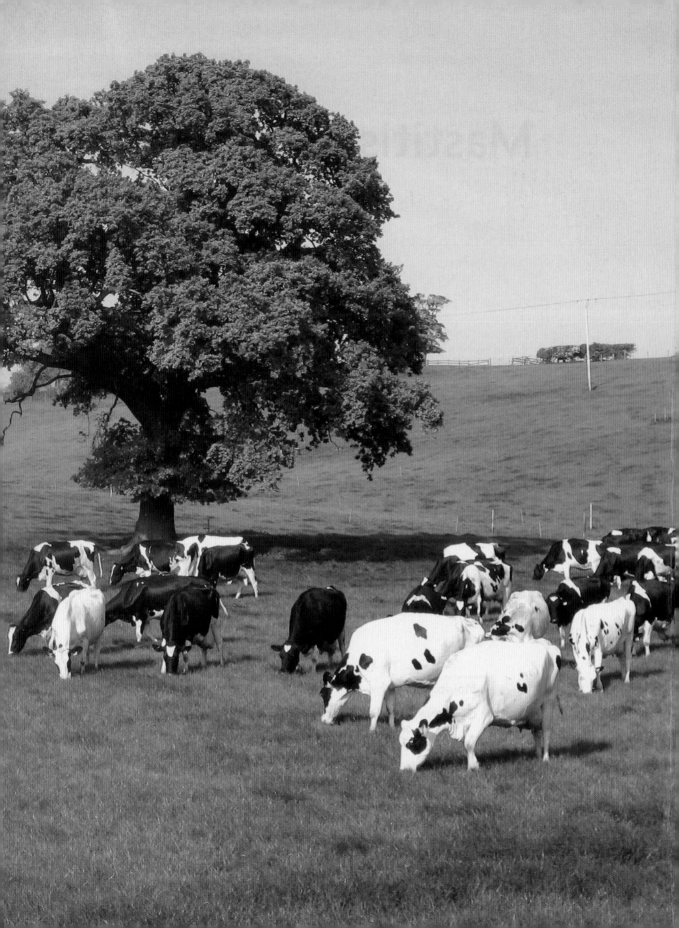

Mastitis in Cattle

Andrew Biggs

THE CROWOOD PRESS

First published in 2009 by
The Crowood Press Ltd
Ramsbury, Marlborough
Wiltshire SN8 2HR

www.crowood.com

British Library Cataloguing-in-Publication Data
A catalogue record for this book is available from the British Library.

ISBN 978 1 84797 071 8

Frontispiece: Bluebells.

Typeset by Bookcraft, Stroud, Gloucestershire
Printed and bound in Malaysia by Times Offset (M) Sdn Bhd

Contents

Abbreviations

ABW acid boiling wash
ACR automatic cluster remover
ADAS Agricultural Development and Advisory Service
ADF Assured Dairy Farms (formerly NDFAS, *vide infra*)
AI artificial insemination
AMC automatic milk conductivity
AMS automatic milking system; Automatic Milking Systems
ANSI apparent new sub-clinical infection
BHM bovine herpes mamillitis
BMSCC bulk milk somatic cell count
BSE bovine spongiform encephalopathy
BT bluetongue
BVD bovine virus diarrhoea
cfu colony-forming unit
CIS Cattle Information Service
CMT California Milk Test
CNS Coagulase-negative *Staphylococci*
CVL Central Veterinary Laboratory
DCT dry cow therapy
ET embryo transfer
EU European Union
FAWC Farm Animal Welfare Council
FMD foot-and-mouth disease
GBS [Lancefield's] Group B *Streptococcus*
HSCC high somatic cell count
IMI intramammary infection
ISQT intermittent serial quarter testing
MAA milk amyloid A
MAFF Ministry of Agriculture, Fisheries, and Food

MDC Milk Development Council
MIC minimum inhibitory concentration
MLST multi-locus sequence typing
MMB Milk Marketing Board
MRL maximum residue limit
NDFAS National Dairy Farm Assured Scheme
NEB negative energy balance
NIRD National Institute for Research into Dairying
NMC National Mastitis Council
NML National Milk Laboratories
NMR National Milk Records
NSAID non-steroidal anti-inflammatory drugs
PCR polymerase chain reaction
PFGE pulsed-field gel electrophoresis
PMTD post-milking teat disinfection
PrMTD pre-milking teat disinfection
RAPD random amplified polymorphic DNA
REA restriction enzyme analysis
RFLP random fragment length polymorphism
SCC somatic cell count
SIM [media] sulphide production, indole production and motility
SUAM *Streptococcus uberis* adhesion molecule
TB [bovine] tuberculosis
TBC total bacterial count
TCI Teat Club International
TVC total viable count
VLA Veterinary Laboratories Agency
WBC white blood cell

Dedication

Dedicated to my sister Alison, who sadly passed away
during the writing of this book.

Acknowledgements

This book has developed in my mind over many years and draws on both personal experience and that of friends and colleagues involved with mastitis from around the world, including other veterinary surgeons, research workers and farmers. I am grateful to the Teat Club International, the Institute for Animal Health and in particular to Martin Shearn and Eric Hillerton for allowing me to use images from their photograph library. I am also grateful to Keith Cutler for reviewing the book so ably and to Mandy Boddy for help and advice on the laboratory work. I would like to thank those farmers who have given me the opportunity to take numerous photographs, some of which feature in the book. I would also like to thank all those who have helped to make this book possible and, in particular, my wife Vikki for her support, patience and tolerance during this and many other projects.

CHAPTER ONE

What Is Mastitis and Why Does It Matter?

INTRODUCTION

Mastitis is one of the most common and most costly diseases of dairy cattle and can also be a disease of considerable significance in beef cattle. The ubiquitous presence in the farm environment of many of the bacteria commonly associated with mastitis on, in or around the cow means that mastitis cannot be realistically eradicated but more controlled to an acceptable level. Equally, the wide variety of causes of mastitis makes the development of an all-encompassing, multivalent vaccine protecting against all strains of all bacteria known to cause the mastitis, let alone other, less common infectious agents, highly unlikely. It is for these reasons that the continued advancement of our understanding of the processes involved in mastitis and its control and the application of that knowledge in management techniques at a farm level will continue to be of huge importance to the dairy industry.

Mastitis in an individual cow can vary in severity from a mild swollen mammary gland, which may self-cure or respond easily to treatment, to a long-term infection which never really clears up despite treatment, to an extremely sick cow which, on occasion, can result in death. In general terms, milk production is reduced or in some cases lost from an affected mammary gland, which has a profound effect on the economics of the dairy industry by reducing the volume of milk produced which is fit to be sold for human consumption. These losses in production are in part due to the need to discard milk while the cow is under treatment and for a period after treatment, but also from a longer-term effect as milk yields are often reduced in the affected gland following a clinical case of mastitis, as they are on occasion with low-grade and less obvious sub-clinical infections. These longer-term effects in yield and the sometimes repeated mastitis cases can result in the premature culling of the cow. There are, in fact, additional costs to the industry over and above the loss of production in the form of labour to tend to the cow and administer the medicines to treat the mastitis case, as well as the cost of the medicines themselves. This reduction or loss of milk production from affected mammary glands also has an impact in the beef industry by way of reduced growth rates in suckled calves, as well as a reduction in the productive life of the breeding cattle, if they are no longer able to produce sufficient milk to rear a calf.

Mastitis is not a simple disease with one single cause but a more complex disease with no simple solution. Despite this complexity the dairy industry has made significant improvements in milk quality, in both hygiene and constituents, as well as reducing both mastitis disease prevalence (the number of infected mammary glands on any one day) and incidence (the number of mastitis cases over a period of time, say one year – often known as the mastitis rate). The incidence of mastitis in the United Kingdom over the last forty years,

Clinical mastitis cases
(per 100 cows per year)

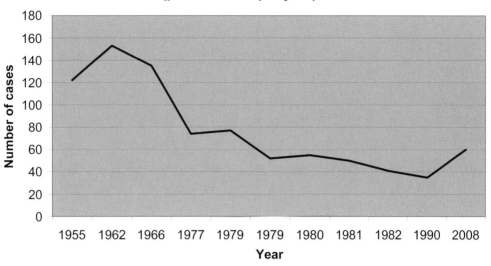

Improvement in mastitis rates in the United Kingdom over the last fifty years.

as measured by clinical mastitis rates in dairy cattle, has dropped from approximately 150 cases per 100 cows per year in the 1960s, to a low of thirty to forty cases per 100 cows per year in the late 1990s.

In recent years the improvements in clinical mastitis rates has reached a plateau and some data indicate that there has, in fact, been a slight upturn in both mastitis prevalence and incidence. These data are complicated by a number of factors which will cause variation in both the interpretation and accuracy of the quoted figures; however, the increases in herd size and milk yield within the industry may well be playing a part in the suggested increase in mastitis rates. Mastitis rates obtained from farm records will be influenced by the fact that clinical mastitis is generally farmer-diagnosed and -recorded. Clinical mastitis detection rates will be affected by an individual farmer's diagnostic criteria, which may result in under- or over-recording, while the record accuracy will depend on the diligence with which the records are kept; incomplete records would lead to an underestimate of case incidence.

The drive by legislation to improve milk quality, facilitated by financial penalties for poor milk quality, coupled with a greater understanding of infection dynamics has led to a move towards the early treatment of mastitis to the point that sub-clinical cases are now often being treated, as opposed to the more common scenario of just clinical cases receiving treatment. This will inevitably, at least initially, have an upward influence on the mastitis treatment rate and may go some way to explaining why the reduction in reported mastitis rates has ceased and may even be increasing slightly. However, early treatment of infection in this way will reduce the duration of intramammary infections, which, in turn, will reduce the chance of spread of contagious pathogens to other cows or quarters in the herd, and, if done in a logical and selective manner, would be expected to result in a downward influence on mastitis rates.

Measurement of prevalence is less simple, particularly as some mastitis infections are hidden (sub-clinical) and not obvious to the naked eye. The dairy industry worldwide has

9

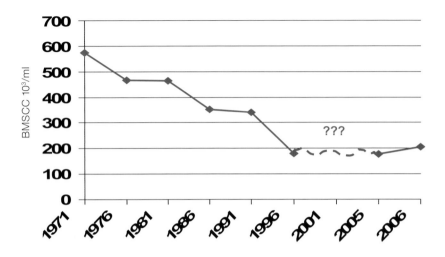

Improvement in BMSCC in England and Wales over the last thirty-five years.

for some years used an indirect measure of infection to assess the prevalence of mastitis at a herd level and used this for quality monitoring and payment purposes. The mastitis prevalence, particularly of sub-clinical mastitis, can be inferred by measuring the somatic cell count (SCC or inflammatory white blood cells) in milk. Similar reductions to those seen in clinical mastitis have taken place over the last forty years and bulk milk somatic cell count (BMSCC) have dropped from 573,000 cells/ml in 1971 to approximately 200,000 cells/ml.

Recent data for England and Wales can be found on the MDC Datum website: www.mdcdatum.org.uk/MilkSupply/milkquality.html. Much of this improvement has been driven by a better understanding of the disease and, in particular, the development of the NIRD five-point plan in the mid 1960s. This five-point plan aimed to reduce the prevalence of mastitis-causing bacteria on farms and minimize the spread of pathogens from cow to cow. Uptake by farmers was variable and, by 1990, approximately twenty-five years after it was developed, only one-third of farmers were using all five recommended practices.

Farming has always adapted to changing times and dairy farming is no exception. There has been a continual reduction in the number of dairy herds in the United Kingdom while those herds remaining have increased in size (number of cows) and milk production (yield). This steady exodus of herds from the industry has resulted in a reduction from approximately 106,000 holdings, with an average herd size of fifteen cows fifty years ago, to the 2007 situation of 17,846 holdings in the United Kingdom, with an average of nearly ninety cows producing a total of 13.5 billion litres of milk. England and Wales now has less than 12,500 dairy farms and the relatively unchanged exodus of between 6 and 6.5 per cent of dairy farms a year continues.

This trend is seen throughout the European Union (EU). As a consequence of these changes there has been a move towards larger, commercially-run businesses, rather than small family-run farms. This continual change seen in the nature of dairy farms of increasing herd size and production is driven by economies of scale and efficiency, but there have also been influences from changes in the industry itself. The introduction of payment schemes based on milk quality and hygiene has improved the product but has possibly accelerated the exodus of some farmers from the industry. Other factors affecting

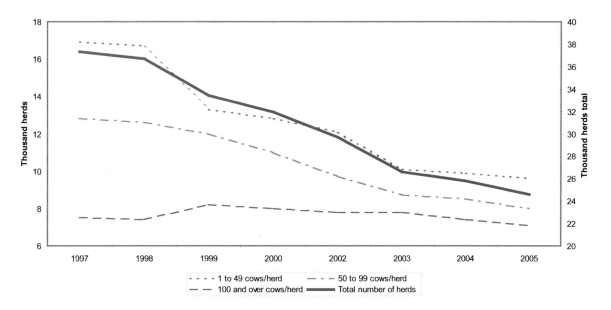

Trends in total UK dairy herds highlighting the reduction in the number of smaller herds. Source: DEFRA. Reproduced by permission of DairyCo, formerly the Milk Development Council, and Eurostat.

Dairy industry EU. Farm data – Number of EU dairy farmers (deliveries + direct sales)

	1998	1999	2000	2001	2002	2003	2004*	2005*
Germany	163,600	142,900	129,892	125,100	119,800	117,100	115,200	112,000
France	140,354	134,394	128,500	123,720	119,497	115,034	109,900*	105,500*
Italy	90,601	80,885	74,457	63,090	59,995	57,358	55,000*	48,200*
Netherlands	37,160	35,421	33,274	25,985	24,775	23,864	23,000*	22,200*
Belgium	18,919	18,477	17,639	17,942	17,154	16,571	15,817	14,500*
Luxembourg	1,261	1,230	1,165	1,112	1,081	1,026	1,006	990
United Kingdom	35,588	34,553	25,853	25,779	22,876	21,383	19,300*	17,800*
Irish Republic	32,856	32,475	29,076	27,814	26,598	25,212	23,800	22,400
Denmark	11,373	10,570	9,737	9,737	8,062	7,400	6,600	5,950
Greece	15,460	13,916	12,435	11,031	9,637	8,655	7,600*	6,800*
Spain	74,230	64,776	56,379	50,362	45,905	41,149	37,300*	31,100*
Portugal	40,832	31,558	23,869	20,588	19,174	17,461	16,027	14,700*
Austria	72,148	72,358	63,949	61,191	60,786	57,268	51,031	50,000
Finland	28,233	26,195	22,225	20,731	19,416	18,143	16,928	15,862
Sweden	14,174	13,243	12,168	11,299	10,557	9,853	9,200	8,700
EU-15	776,789	712,951	640,618	595,481	656,313	537,477	507,709*	476,702*

*December census.

Reproduced by permission of DairyCo, formerly the Milk Development Council, and Eurostat.

production and economics in the last twenty years, such as the introduction of milk quotas in 1984, bovine spongiform encephalopathy (BSE), the spread of bovine tuberculosis (TB) to non-endemic areas, foot-and-mouth disease in 2001 and 2007, and bluetongue BTV8 in 2007 and 2008, and threats of BTV1 and BTV4, have all had significant effects on the industry. Nevertheless, mastitis still remains a costly and important disease to the UK dairy farmer.

WHAT IS MASTITIS?

Mastitis is generally the result of the invasion and establishment of infectious agents within the mammary gland; however, its occurrence can be greatly influenced by a variety of factors. It is best seen as an interrelationship between the host (the cow), the pathogen (most commonly bacteria) and the environment (which can influence both the cows and the pathogen).

Often control measures are directed at the management factors which are known to influence new infection rates, and these will

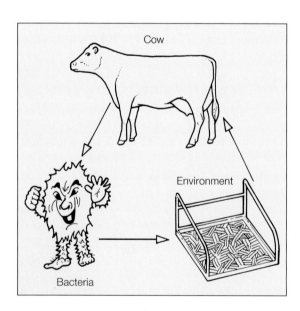

Mastitis triangle – a balance between cow, bacteria and the environment.

vary from pathogen to pathogen. As a consequence, there are many and sometimes conflicting control measures advocated for mastitis control. It is this complex nature, in part at least, which causes mastitis to remain a major problem in both beef and dairy cows.

Definition

The word mastitis literally means inflammation of the mammary gland and is derived from *mast*, the breast, and *itis*, meaning inflammation. The inflammation is most commonly a pathophysiological response to the invasion and multiplication of micro-organisms, usually bacteria, but it could also be caused by chemical, thermal or mechanical injury. The inflammation results in a range of physical and chemical changes in the milk and pathological changes in the udder tissue. Although the topic is covered in more detail later in the book, mastitis can be divided into two broad categories: clinical, where changes to the milk, udder and sometimes the cow can be detected with the naked eye, or sub-clinical, where the changes can be more subtle and laboratory tests are needed to detect it.

Effects

Mastitis can cause changes in milk composition and yield, the udder and even the cow. The degree to which these changes occur in individual cows can vary considerably and will depend on pathogen factors, such as the severity and duration of the infection, as well as the causative micro-organisms; host factors such as the nutritional or immune status of the cow, as well as the milk production of the cow; and environmental factors such as the ambient temperature, humidity or cleanliness. In severe cases a mastitis infection can become systemic and affect the cow resulting in a range of clinical signs such as an elevated temperature, inappetence, general malaise; severe cases may lead to diarrhoea, dehydration and ultimately the death of the cow.

Mastitis is almost exclusively caused by bacteria, some of which can produce toxins that can directly damage the milk-producing

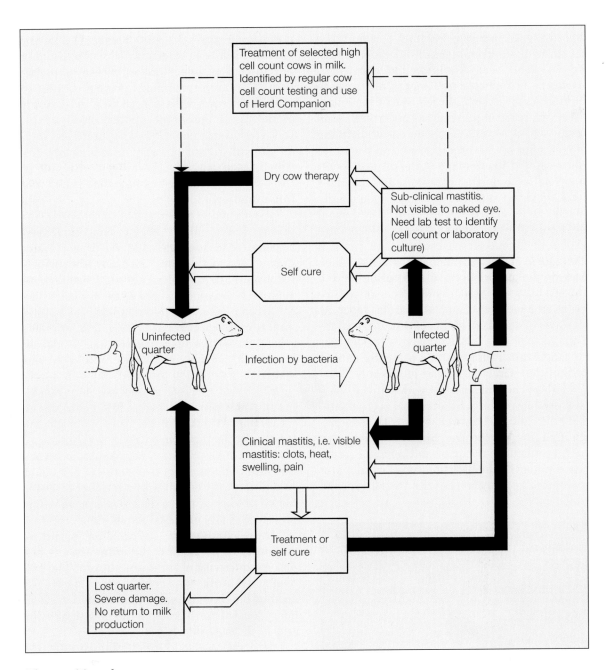

The mastitis cycle.

secretory tissue of the mammary gland. The presence of the bacteria will generally initiate an inflammatory response within the mammary tissue in an attempt to eliminate the invading micro-organisms. This inflammatory response results in the production of chemical mediators and inflammatory proteins which amplify the host response and, in part, are also responsible for the decreased milk production and the compositional changes seen in milk from infected quarters and cows. The end result is an accompanying inflammation leading to an increase in somatic cells in the mastitic milk and changes in the udder resulting in pain, heat, swelling and sometimes hardness or induration. There is an increase in blood-derived somatic cell, including leucocytes (white blood cells such as neutrophils and lymphocytes) as well as the increased shedding of epithelial-derived somatic cells in the milk. As a result of the damage to the normal secretory epithelium, the compositional changes tend to be an increase in blood components in the milk and a decrease in the normal milk constituents. Some of these changes are visible to the naked eye, notably the physical changes in the appearance of the milk, which include flakes or clots, discoloration and a change to a more serous consistency or watery milk, whereas the chemical changes, such as changes in the proportions of protein, sodium and chloride ions, or the changes in lactoferrin and other inflammatory proteins, cannot be detected without analysis of the milk.

Changes in milk quality with clinical mastitis are more marked than those seen in sub-clinical mastitis; however, even with sub-clinical mastitis the changes can be significant in both economic and nutritional terms. Protein content may be unchanged overall in sub-clinical mastitis, but the changes in the types of

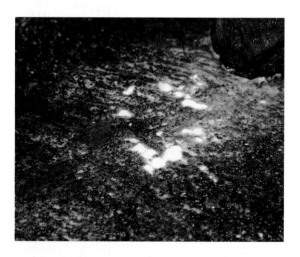

Mastitis clots stripped out of an affected quarter on to concrete standing.

protein present are significant. The major protein in milk is casein, which is both highly nutritious and important in cheese manufacture. The often unchanged protein content of milk from cows with a high SCC is a result of increased but lower quality blood serum proteins often known as whey proteins, such as serum albumen and immunoglobulins which leach out into the milk as a result of the destructive processes associated with the inflammation.

This damage making the epithelial membrane leaky also allows the increased passage of sodium, chloride and bicarbonate. Conversely, potassium, normally the principal mineral in milk, declines slightly due to its leakage between damaged secretory cells into the lymph. Calcium, perhaps the best known mineral associated with milk but, in fact, second in terms of concentration, is closely bound with casein, and interference in casein synthesis results in reduced calcium levels in milk from cows with mastitis. As a result, many veterinary surgeons will administer intravenous calcium as part of the treatment for cows suffering from a case of toxic mastitis. However, the association between hypocalcaemia and toxic mastitis is one of lowered blood calcium, often resulting in recumbency (milk fever) predisposing to mastitis, rather than an effect of the mastitis per se. As a result of all these changes in the principal constituents and, in particular, the minerals, the pH and conductivity of milk are altered. The pH of normal milk is generally slightly acid at around 6.6, but increases commonly to 6.8 or 6.9 in mastitic milk and may on occasions even approach neutrality at 7.0.

Further consequences of the damaged blood–milk barrier result as enzymes, from cells damaged by the inflammatory process, leak from the blood into the milk. The most notable is lipase, which will break down milk fats to free fatty acids, resulting in the off-tastes of rancid milk and can also inhibit starter cultures for cheese or yoghurt. Plasmin, another enzyme which attacks casein, will further reduce casein levels in mastitic milk and also significantly

reduce cheese yields and yields of other manufactured milk products. Normal milk is isotonic
with blood and, due to the presence of lactose,
lower concentrations of sodium and chloride
are needed in milk to compensate for the presence of lactose. However, in mastitis, when
lactose levels fall due to reduced synthesis, deg-
radation and leakage to the blood, the sodium
and chloride levels rise to maintain isotonicity
with blood, and it is for this reason that mastitic milk can have a slightly salty taste. The
net effect is increased milk conductivity, which
has been used for mastitis diagnosis.

WHY DOES MASTITIS MATTER?

Welfare
The Farm Animal Welfare Council (FAWC),
the independent advisory body established by
the British government in 1979, state that,
'The welfare of an animal includes its physical and mental state and we consider that
good animal welfare implies both fitness and
a sense of well-being.' They have provided a
framework to define ideal states that are applicable to all animal production systems termed
the 'Five Freedoms'. The third freedom states,
'Freedom from pain, injury or disease'.

There is no question that clinical mastitis
is a painful condition and in very severe cases
cows will appear very sick and distressed.
However, research has shown that, even in
relatively mild cases, cows show a reduced
threshold for pain, indicating that pain can be
a significant consequence for a cow suffering
from a case of clinical mastitis. This reduced
pain threshold persisted until the fourth day
in mild cases, but could last as long as twenty
days in severe cases. Veterinary surgeons
often use analgesics, such as non-steroidal
anti-inflammatory drugs (NSAID) in more
acute cases. These drugs are strong pain
relievers and have antipyretic (help to reduce
a fever) and anti-inflammatory properties, as
well as having an added benefit of protecting
the cow to some extent from the toxic effects
that some bacterial infections induce, known
as an anti-endotoxic effect.

Food Quality and Safety
Mastitis has a variety of effects on the constituents of milk and many of these effects have
implications for the food industry. Changes in
milk quality associated with sub-clinical mastitis can have significant effects on keeping
quality and cheese yield. Somatic cells that
are present in milk during an infection are
involved in the conversion of plasminogen
to plasmin. Plasmin is a proteolytic enzyme,
produced by the cow, which can break down
casein and decrease cheese yield. Decreased
cheese yield, when milk SCC is high, is caused
by an increased loss of casein and fat into whey
during cheese-making.

Although milk has the potential to harbour
pathogens harmful to human health, the vast
majority of reported cases of milk-related
human illness are linked to the contamination of the milk after harvesting from the cow,
or from cases within the small proportion of
the population who drink unpasteurized milk.
Tuberculosis is perhaps the best known infection historically linked to drinking raw milk.
However, the Defra zoonosis report 2001 states
that it is important to note that human tuberculosis is usually caused by *Mycobacterium
tuberculosis* (by and large usually acquired
from another human) and not *Mycobacterium
bovis*, which is the cause of bovine tuberculosis.
Mycobacterium bovis infection was formerly
an important zoonotic disease and at that
time was most often transmitted to man by
milk. The advent of pasteurization and a com-
pulsory eradication programme in cattle had
significantly reduced human infection with
this organism from the levels recorded prior
to the 1950s. In England and Wales in 2001
there were twenty-seven laboratory reports of
tuberculosis in humans due to *Mycobacterium
bovis*. None of the cases in 2001 had a known
current link with disease in cattle. More
recently, the bovine tuberculosis eradication policy of the 1950s has been downgraded
to a control programme in recognition that
eradication is not currently possible. Figures
are now back up to the pre-eradication levels,
with nearly 30,000 cattle slaughtered in 2005

and 5,500 herds under restriction, as opposed to the near eighty herds under restriction at its lowest point in the early 1980s. Although the risk is low because cattle are removed by a test and cull programme, before the advanced stage of the disease required to progress to excretion in the milk is common, the recent increases do mean we still need to be vigilant as to the potential of this zoonosis.

Economics

Mastitis costs the UK dairy industry approximately £200m and the world cost is estimated to be US $200bn. The financial outlay by the industry as a whole or at the farm level will encompass both treatment and preventive measures, aimed at both clinical and sub-clinical mastitis. The expenditure can be split into investment into preventive measures, which will be aiming for a return on investment, and treatment expenditure, which will be a less certain investment aimed at limiting the financial losses. It is well recognized that some preventive measures will have a high return on investment while others will not. Equally, treatment of cases of mastitis that have a good chance of success will be better value for money than attempting to treat cases where

success is very unlikely and culling is a more sensible option.

Both clinical and sub-clinical mastitis have an economic impact on the dairy industry. The industry has always recognized the economic impact of clinical mastitis, where the cost is easier to calculate than with sub-clinical mastitis, because more of the direct costs are identifiable; however, there is always a yield and quality effect that has to be estimated. In spite of this, the industry for many years was not receptive to the idea of 'hidden' losses from sub-clinical mastitis, and calculations indicating a reduction in yield were not well received. *See* table opposite and graph below.

Calculations of mastitis costs can be broadly split into direct and indirect costs, but even these categories have a degree of overlap when looking at definitions by a number of workers. The costs associated with clinical mastitis are easier to calculate, with the direct costs being the most simple to quantify. Generally, direct costs will be those that can be attributed to the mastitis (the clinical case in the instance of clinical mastitis), whereas indirect costs are those incurred as a result of, or subsequent to, the mastitis. There are also significant costs to the industry of on-going preventive measures.

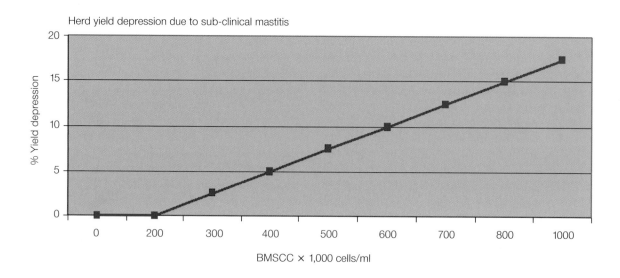

Reduction of milk yield with increasing bulk milk somatic cell count.

Herd infection prevalence and production loss with increasing BMSCC

Bulk tank SCC/ml	% infected quarters	% production loss
200,000	5	0
300,000	10	2.5
400,000	15	5.0
500,000	20	7.5
1,000,000	35	20
1,500,000	50	32.5

It would seem obvious that the overall costs of preventive management measures are spread over the whole herd, as are the benefits. However, it may not be so obvious that the effects of a successful treatment of a single infected quarter are not restricted to the cow under treatment alone. Increasingly, the importance is becoming recognized that the removal by successful treatment of an infected quarter from a herd reduces the chance of spread within the herd, thus benefiting the herd and not only the cow under treatment. This has historically been better recognized when considering the benefits to the herd of culling a cow with a persistent, non-responsive infection. This benefit to the other cows will be more significant when contagious bacteria are involved since it is in this situation that there will be more likelihood that the removal of the infected quarter will reduce the chance of new infections in other quarters, either in that cow or other cows. Environmentally-derived infections tend to be shorter lived, rarely spread from cow to cow, and the environmental source of the infection is unaffected by successful elimination of an infection from an infected quarter, and so the treatment benefits will tend to be less to the herd and effectively limited to the infected cow.

Advances in the computer-aided analysis and interpretation of individual cow SCCs from routine monthly milk-recording data have focused attention on the dynamics of non-clinical intramammary infections and stimulated a move towards the treatment of persistent sub-clinical mastitis, and, in particular, those cases identified as recently acquired persistent infection as these will have a greater chance of being successfully treated (*see* Herd Companion, Chapter 5). The rationale for this move to treating selected sub-clinical infections is based on the benefits accruing to the herd by removing potentially contagious infections as soon as they can be identified and before they have a chance to spread. This has tended to blur the accuracy of mastitis rate records as more sub-clinical mastitis is being treated alongside clinical mastitis and will have an effect on both the direct and the indirect costs and benefits associated with the cases being treated.

Clinical Mastitis: Direct Costs

- cow costs
- treatment costs
  - drugs – intramammary tubes (and injections where appropriate)
  - direct labour costs
    herdsperson's time to treat case
    veterinary surgeon's time, if appropriate
- reduced milk sales from discarded milk during treatment and for the withhold period.

Clinical Mastitis: Indirect Costs

- cow costs
  - subsequent yield reduction
  - repeat cases later in lactation
  - predisposition to other diseases
  - direct mortality.increased risk of culling resulting in
  - high replacement rates
  - loss of genetic potential

Calculations to estimate the average cost of a clinical case of mastitis can be made by looking at mild cases (farmer-treated), severe cases (requiring a veterinary surgeon's visit) and fatal cases. The direct costs of each type of treatment can be calculated along with the indirect long-term effects on subsequent production, together with the replacement costs of a proportion of the cows being replaced from early culling in mild and severe cases, as well as the total loss from fatal cases. Once the costs for each type of mastitis are determined these can be weighted by their relative occurrence. It has been estimated that 90 per cent of mastitis treatments are for mild cases, 9.8 per cent for severe cases and 0.2 per cent for fatal cases. Taking the cow costs for clinical mastitis, the direct cost for an average case have been estimated to be from £40 to £50 and the indirect cow costs to be from £140 to £150, giving a total for an average case of mastitis of between £180 and £200.

Sub-clinical Mastitis: Direct Costs

Direct costs attributable to an increased BMSCC are perhaps the most obvious cost to farmers other than the cost of treating clinical cases and these take the form of payment penalties. Different payment penalties in pence per litre (ppl) are levied on individual farms by first-time buyers, but are generally triggered by a BMSCC >200,000 cells/ml. These penalties are generally banded, becoming more significant with increasing BMSCC and represent approximately between <1 and 5 per cent of milk value, depending on the milk contract and the BMSCC level.

The introduction of variable milk pricing based on quality in the United Kingdom in the mid 1990s put a spotlight on the economics of sub-clinical mastitis and the trend of reducing BMSCC was significantly accelerated during this period (*see* graph on page 10). As a result of EU directive 92/46/EC, an upper ceiling of 400,000 cells/ml was placed on milk produced for human consumption within the European Union. The figures used around the world for upper BMSCC limits for milk sold for human consumption vary, although both New Zealand and Australia use the 400,000 cells/ml upper limit. Canada uses 500,000 cells/ml as the upper limit, while it is interesting to note that in many states in the USA an upper limit of 750,000 cells/ml is still applicable, despite several discussions within the industry over recent years and many US herds achieving a BMSCC similar to that in other major dairying countries of the world. In the United Kingdom significant financial penalties were used as an 'incentive' to encourage compliance and these penalties could exceed one-third of the milk price. This created an unsustainable financial penalty which no dairy farmer could survive and rapidly encouraged the UK dairy industry to reduce the BMSCC to below 400,000 cells/ml. It has to be said that this was achieved partly by improvements in those herds which remained in the industry, but also by the many dairy farmers unable to make the investments required leaving the industry.

Sub-clinical Mastitis: Indirect Costs

Research has shown that a reduction in yield of 2.5 per cent for every 100,000 cells/ml the BMSCC increased over a threshold of 200,000 cells/ml, can be expected.

Further indirect costs
- herd effects
  - spread to other cows
  - increased herd clinical incidence
  - reduced herd yield from increased risk of sub-clinical infection
- financial penalty effects
  - potential effect on BMSCC once milk returned to the bulk tank
    transient if recovery not complete and SCC still elevated
    permanent if recovery not achieved and infection remains sub-clinical with raised SCC
- potential effect on Bactoscan
- potential to cause an antibiotic milk failure which has significant economic impact

Preventive Management Costs

- labour: time involved in:
  - maintaining general hygiene of cow accommodation
  - good milking routine
  - monthly routine milk recording
  - maintaining accurate clinical and drying off records
  - action lists from analysing and interpreting SCC and clinical records
- consumables
  - teat preparation material (paper towels/medicated towels, etc.)
- teat dip/spray – post-milking (and pre-milking where appropriate)
- dairy chemicals for cleaning parlour (and cluster disinfection where appropriate)
- dry cow preparations
    antibiotic dry cow tubes
    teat sealant internal/external

The economic impacts of mastitis on the dairy herd are many, varied and significant.

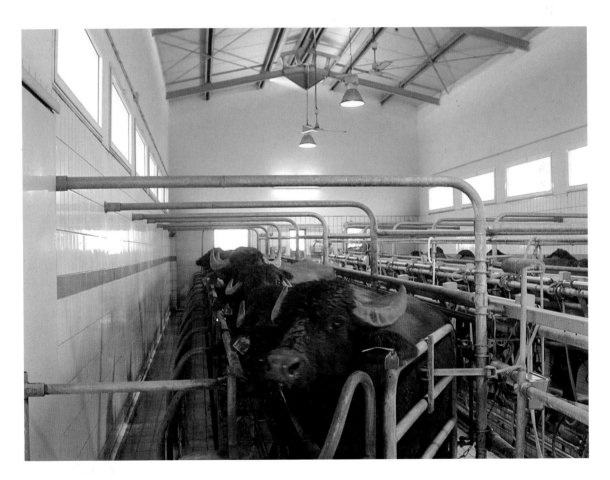

Buffalo being milked.

CHAPTER TWO

Udder and Teat Structure and Function

MILK PRODUCTION OVERVIEW

The mammary gland is a unique organ to mammals and has evolved to nourish the newborn young. In the dairy cow, with the help of modern milking equipment and advances in genetic selection, milk production is far in excess of the requirements of the neonate calf and, in reality, in excess of the original structural design. The increased production and milking machine extraction of milk have resulted in a number of 'production' stresses on the dairy cow's udder. As a consequence of this increased production, the need to fully understand the design and function of the udder and, in particular, the milk secretion and let-down process have been essential in maintaining these increases in dairy cow yields, together with the associated development of the modern milking machine.

The udder of the modern dairy cow has a huge capacity for producing and storing milk. The daily production can be as much as 70ltr in very high-yielding cows, although peak yields of 40 to 50ltr per day would be more common. This would relate to 80 to 90 pint milk bottles produced per day from a cow weighing perhaps 650 to 700kg. This represents a milk production at roughly 7 or 8 per cent of body weight a day for several weeks, almost like you or I metabolically regrowing an arm each day. While it is true that the racehorse is the genuine athlete of the animal kingdom, the dairy cow is the undisputed metabolic athlete.

This high metabolic demand process requires a large supply of nutrients, and it is not surprising that the total udder blood volume for lactating cows is about 8 per cent of the total body blood volume. For a non-lactating cow, udder blood volume is similar at about 7.4 per cent; however, there is a two- to six-fold increase in blood flow in the lactating mammary gland starting two to three days prepartum, and it is this increase in flow that facilitates milk production rather than the volume per se. In a similar fashion, the decrease in production with advancing lactation is not due to decreased blood flow, but it is more due to the loss of secretory epithelial cells through a process of programmed cell death (apoptosis). Nonetheless, a vast supply of nutrients for milk production is essential and 400 to 500ltr of blood will flow through the udder to produce each litre of milk, which in the dairy cow relates to approximately 280ml of blood flow per second. The secretory system within the udder is highly developed and there is also a need for an extensive lymphatic system to help maintain the fluid balance within the udder. When excess fluid accumulation does occur within the tissue spaces this is seen as oedema and can be seen particularly between the udder skin and the udder, increasing the skin thickness such that it can be 'pitted' by digital pressure. Oedema is commonly seen at calving time, and particularly in heifers where the swelling can be seen in front of the udder. (*See* photo on page 182, Chapter 9.)

Milk is produced in the cuboidal epithelial alveolar cells, which are arranged in sacs and surrounded by myoepithelial cells to aid its secretion and transportation via a system of ducts and cisterns for storing the milk, which allows further secretion by reducing back pressure within the alveoli. This storage allows the cow to build up volumes of milk so that it can be released rapidly when the calf suckles or the cow is milked. The milk then travels down ducts to the teat cistern at the base of the udder just above the 'stopcock' of the teat which facilitates this intermittent delivery with its highly sophisticated washer or streak canal in the teat end. The flow down these ducts is facilitated by the contraction of the myoepithelial cells of the alveoli in response to the blood-borne hormone oxytocin, which is released as a consequence of the stimulation of the highly innervated teat and udder skin. It is for this reason that dairy cows should not be stressed or frightened when they enter the milking parlour or the fight and flight hormone adrenalin will inhibit oxytocin release and prevent milk let down. Many dairy farmers will have the radio on not only for their own pleasure but because it is felt that this will mask many of the noises normally associated with a busy milking parlour at milking time and perhaps help to relax the cows ready for milking.

DEVELOPMENT OF THE UDDER

The development of the mammary gland starts early in foetal life and, by the second month of gestation, teat formation has begun. By six months of gestation the udder is almost fully developed, with four separate glands, a median ligament and teat and gland cisterns. The growth of the udder from birth to puberty is at the same pace as the rest of the body (isometric) with some development of the duct system. After puberty growth is more rapid than in the rest of the body (allometric) and the duct system develops further under the influence of oestrogen, with successive oestrus periods (heats). In primaparous (first calving) heifers

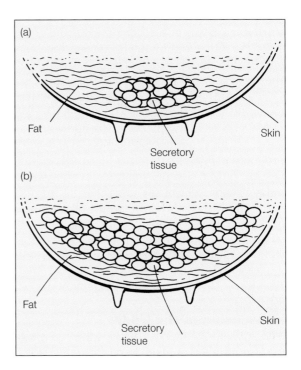

Growth rates and fat deposition in the pubescent udder. (a) High level feeding – average daily gain 1.15kg per day. (b) Moderate level feeding – average daily gain 700g per day.

this growth phase is critical to functional udder development and growth rates of no more than 750g body weight per day will result in less fat and more secretory tissue than growth rates of over 1kg body weight per day.

In early pregnancy the duct system becomes fully formed and canalized. Changes in the mammary gland structure are also seen with multiparous cows between subsequent pregnancies. In the inactive mammary gland, the interstitial spaces between lobes and ducts are filled mainly with fat. There are few alveoli present compared to those in the lactating gland, and the ducts and lobes of the gland are smaller than when the gland is in its active phase. During early pregnancy the epithelial cells of the glandular tissue proliferate rapidly to form the buds which eventually enlarge to form the alveoli. As pregnancy develops, the fat and connective tissue between the lobes and the ducts is replaced by secretory tissue. As the pregnancy advances further, development of the alveoli is influenced by the hormone progesterone. Finally, the secretion of milk is initiated by the rising levels of prolactin late in pregnancy.

The mammary glands are greatly modified and enlarged sweat glands and have a number of features to allow them, in the dairy cow at least, not only to achieve this high level of milk production but also to store it to allow harvesting only twice or sometimes three times a day. The weight of the udder can be significant, particularly when it is full of milk and can be in excess of 50kg. This weight needs to be supported and therefore the udder has to be very well attached to the skeleton and muscles; there are various suspensory ligaments supporting the udder to achieve this.

Suspension of the Udder

The suspensory system of the udder is made up of a number of elastic and fibrous tissues, effectively forming a sling for the udder which imparts a degree of shock-absorbing capacity and also allows the udder to expand as milk accumulates between milkings. The most important structures in this sling are the median and lateral suspensory ligaments; however, other anatomical structures such as the skin and the superficial fascia between the skin and the underlying mammary gland do offer some support.

The anterior (front) edges of the forequarters are attached to the abdominal wall by coarse fibrous tissue, and, although this does not offer major support to the udder, weakening of this attachment can cause the udder to break away from the abdominal wall. This is part of what is referred to as the forequarter attachments when assessing dairy cattle conformation.

The median suspensory ligaments run from their attachment to the abdominal wall as a pair of adjacent, heavy, yellow, elastic sheets of tissue separating the udder into left and right halves. They are reflected underneath

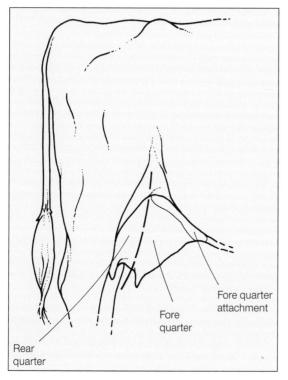

Udder attachment.

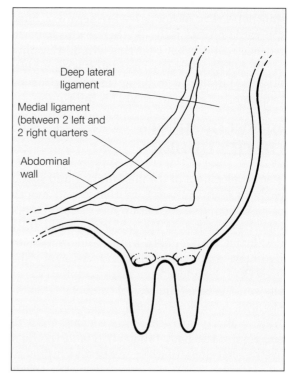

Support of the udder.

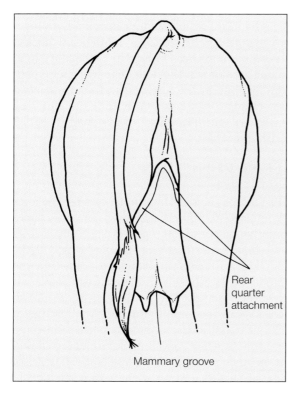

Rear
quarter
attachment

Mammary groove

Udder attachment.

the udder and terminate at the base of the teats, helping to form the natural cleavage of the intermammary groove, having fanned out to cover the underside of the udder, where they meet the lateral suspensory ligaments. The median suspensory ligaments have great tensile strength and are able to give a little as the gland fills with milk to allow for the increased weight of the gland.

The lateral suspensory ligaments have a distinct superficial and deep portion. The superficial layers are mostly fibrous, with less elastic component than the median suspensory ligaments. They run from the pelvic bone, extending downwards and spreading out over the external surface of the udder. The deep layers also originate from the pelvic bone but are thicker and more fibrous and, as they spread out over the convex surface of the udder and almost envelop it, they also have numerous lamellar plates which interdigitate into the glandular tissue. In this way collectively, the lateral suspensory ligaments

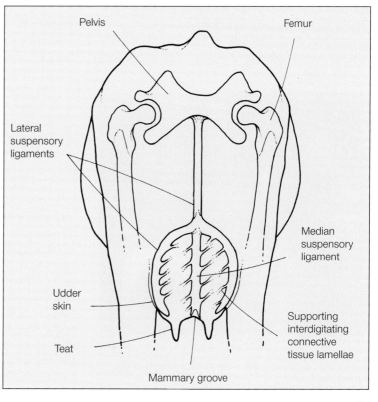

Pelvis

Femur

Lateral
suspensory
ligaments

Median
suspensory
ligament

Udder
skin

Supporting
interdigitating
connective
tissue lamellae

Teat

Mammary groove

Suspensory ligaments supporting the udder.

provide substantial support for the udder. The left and the right lateral suspensory ligament do not join under the bottom of the udder but merge with the median ligament. Their fibrous nature means that, unlike the median ligament, they do not stretch as the gland fills with milk, causing the centre of the udder to pull away from the body as the gland fills.

The suspensory apparatus can break down gradually over time as a result of normal wear and tear. However, premature breakdown of the various parts of the suspensory apparatus can occur from over-engorgement, particularly around the time of calving or as a result of poor udder conformation, which, in this instance, refers to poor udder attachment.

Disruption of the median ligaments will tend to result in the loss of the natural cleavage, allowing the teats to splay out. This can make the cow difficult to milk due to the angle and position of the teats and, on occasion, farmers have been know to add extensions to the short milk tubes to facilitate milking. As a result of the teat angles the condition will predispose the cow to liner slip and impacts, making mastitis infections more common.

Disruption of the lateral ligaments usually involves both deep and superficial parts and

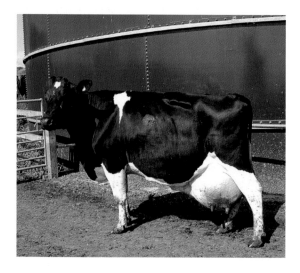

Cow with 'dropped udder' from disruption of the lateral ligaments.

results in the whole udder's dropping, giving a status often referred to as 'teats below hocks'. In severe instances of lateral suspensory ligament breakdown the udder can become so pendulous that, as the cow walks, she cannot avoid knocking it with her feet making the gait very awkward and effectively plays 'keepie uppie' with her udder.

TEAT FUNCTION

The teat is the only functional exit for the milk from each gland and, although generally there is only one per gland, up to 50 per cent of cows will have supernumerary teats of which a proportion will communicate with the normal gland while others will have a very small but separate gland. On occasions, these small glands can succumb to infection and produce a classic mastitic discharge which has no bearing on the adjacent main milk-producing gland. It is also possible for these supernumerary teats to act as a route of entry into the normal mammary gland, predisposing these glands to mastitis and, as a consequence, it is common practice to remove them at a few weeks old.

The role of the teat is to supply milk on demand for the suckling calf while resisting the ingress of bacteria to infect that milk supply. However, unless the teat becomes erect and turgid, the milk would not flow into it and a flaccid teat will not allow the calf to effectively suckle. The teat is richly innervated and, as a consequence, can feed back the stimuli of the calf suckling to the brain, which facilitates further milk let down via oxytocin release. It is for this reason that stimulation of the teats and udder before the milking machine unit is attached is essential to encourage early milk let down. If this is not accomplished or if the cow is nervous and milk let down does not occur, then delayed let down may occur from residual oxytocin (which has a 1½ to 2min half life), or a secondary release of oxytocin may occur; but either way there will be an initial flow of cisternal milk followed by a break in the milk flow before the milk let down makes the milk from higher in the udder available

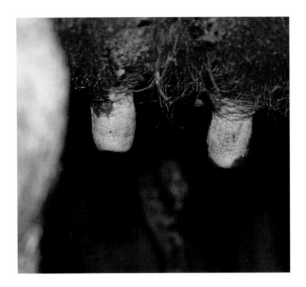

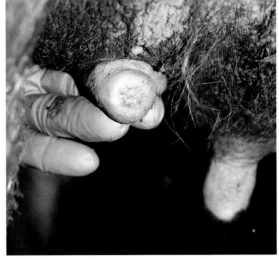

Short, flat-ended teats are more prone to mastitis.

and flow returns. This is sometimes referred to as bimodal milk let down or bimodal milk flow. Milk let down can be both unconditioned in response to these types of stimulus or, particularly in the dairy cow, conditioned in response to the routine and sounds of the milking process.

TEAT STRUCTURE

Teat size and shape vary with those from the cranial (front) glands tending to be longer (average length approximately 6.5cm and just under 3cm in diameter) than those from the caudal (rear) glands (average length approximately 5.2cm and 2.6cm in diameter), despite the fact that the yields are greater from the caudal glands. Some teats are conical with quite pointed teat ends, while others are more cylindrical with slab sides, but still with a rounded base; it is thought that these are less prone to mastitis. Teats with flat or inverted bases seem to be associated with larger diameter streak canals and are more prone to mastitis.

The teat skin is thin and has no hair, sweat glands nor sebaceous glands, which makes it very prone to drying out, which is why much effort is taken to keep teat skin moisturized

with emollients and humectants, which are included for this purpose in post-milking teat disinfectant dips and sprays. Despite being thin, the skin has a thick, keratinized epidermal (outer) layer covering the normal squamous cell epithelium, which helps with waterproofing and is a deterrent to bacterial growth. The word 'keratin' comes from the Greek *keratos* meaning horn. Keratin is a fibrous, structural protein of hair, nails, horn, hooves, wool, feathers and skin. A quarter of the amino acids in keratin are cystine, whose ability to form strong bridging (disulphide) bonds with other cystine units accounts for keratin's great stability. The infiltration of the outer layers of the teat epithelium with keratin affords a strengthening and rigidity which helps the teat resist the forces encountered when a calf suckles or when a cow is milked by machine. To help the rigidity of the teat structure there are fingers (papillae) of epidermal tissue that interdigitate with the deeper dermis. The dermis contains elastic connective tissue with blood vessels and nerves which infiltrate the epidermis, and two layers of muscle tissue (an inner layer of longitudinal muscles and an outer layer of circular muscles). The innermost layer lining the lumen of the teat (the teat cistern) is similar to the lining of the gland cistern and the ducts draining the mammary gland lobes. It is formed by a double layer of cuboidal epithelium, which acts as the barrier between the milk and the blood and the blood immune products, such as white blood cells (WBCs), acute phase proteins, such as lactoferrin, and other immune chemical mediators. These palisades of brick-like cells are joined by tight cell junctions which prevent leakage between the cells. However, these tight junctions can become permeable rather than physically separated as a result of an inflammatory process, such as mastitis or in response to high doses of oxytocin. The sudden increase in WBCs in milk is an important defensive mechanism and, if the inflammation causes damage to the epithelium, the movement of inflammatory products will increase significantly. A practical outcome of this is that the cow's SCC will rise dramatically.

The teat cistern ends at the teat or streak canal through which the milk is removed by a suckling calf or milking machine. Just at the transition between the teat cistern and the streak canal there is a collection of folds of the epithelium (Furstenberg's rosette) which don't seem to have a mechanical function in preventing the leakage of milk. However, the increased epithelial surface area may help in increasing the ability to recruit protective WBCs and may act as a 'gatekeeper', helping to prevent a higher invasion of mastitis-causing bacteria.

Teat or Streak Canal

At the end of the teat is the streak canal which is the functional barrier between the, hopefully, clean, uninfected, internal milk secretory system of the mammary gland and the potentially dirty, external environment. The streak canal is the main barrier against intramammary infection. Although a very small part of the cow, it has enormous importance in terms of the long-term viability of a dairy cow. If the teat end itself is damaged this defence mechanism is compromised and the normal effectiveness of the function of the streak canal is all too obviously reduced as mastitis is an almost inevitable consequence. This can also be important during the treatment of

mastitis where only the tip of an intramammary tube should be inserted (partial insertion technique) to avoid damaging the streak canal and removing the all-important keratin lining. *See* photos on page 170, Chapter 7.

The teat or streak canal is lined with stratified squamous epithelium identical to that of skin and is, in fact, continuous with that of the outer teat skin. This change from the double cuboidal epithelium of the teat cistern occurs at Furstenberg's rosette. The continual desquamation of the surface results in the formation of keratin, which has antibacterial properties and may also block the canal between milkings, acting as a barrier to penetration by bacteria. If this keratin is lost, either by the shearing forces of milk flow flushing it out during milking or by the damage caused by introducing the nozzle of an intramammary treatment tube, the barrier effect is lessened and the streak canal is less resistant to bacterial invasion, with a case of mastitis being a more likely outcome.

The streak canal is effectively kept closed by sphincter muscles around the canal, although the pressure to penetrate it can be measured and will vary with lactational age, stage of lactation and time after milking. When a cow is milked the sphincter muscles relax, allowing the orifice to open and milk to pass. The streak canal remains open for 20 to 30min after milking and this increases the chance of bacteria penetrating the canal and gaining entry to the gland, and the possibility of setting up an infection which, if not eliminated, may well result in a case of mastitis. Post-milking teat disinfection is aimed at helping to minimize the chance of bacteria gaining access to the gland after milking. Additionally, keeping cows standing for 20min to half an hour after milking, by, for example, providing access to fresh feed, also helps minimize teat-end contamination before the streak canal closes again. Cows with weak, relaxed or incompetent circular smooth muscle are called 'fast milkers'. They have leaky streak canals and may well milk out in the parlour in 2 or 3min but will be more prone to mastitis. Cows with tight circular smooth muscle are called 'hard milkers' and may take 10min or more to milk because the milk will be expressed as a fine spray and the milk flow is very slow. Although the relationship is not clear, it also appears that fast milkers tend to be higher yielding cows, however, it is not clear whether this is causal.

The streak canal has an equally important role in protecting the mammary gland during the dry period (non-lactating period) when the epidermal tissue lining the streak canal forms an effective keratin plug. However, work from New Zealand and the United Kingdom shows that there is a large variation in the proportion of cows which do form an effective keratin plug, and those cows that do not are at greater risk of picking up an infection in the dry period. Various research has shown that 50 per cent of teats are still open ten days after drying off, 22 per cent at forty-two days (with a variation of 10 to 33 per cent and with 65 per cent of cows having at least one open teat), but by sixty days after drying off less than 5 per cent of teats are open. 'Open' is defined as when secretion can easily be expressed. In an attempt to help those cows with incomplete keratin plugs, both external (Dry Flex, DeLaval) and internal (Orbeseal Pfizer) teat seals are used to help overcome the patency of the streak canal in these cows.

Microscopic Anatomy of the Udder and Milk Synthesis

The intricate details of the microscopic structure of the secretory tissue within the udder are outwith the scope of this book, but an overview is helpful to understand how it is influenced by mastitis.

As already stated, each of the four quarters functions as an independent gland within the udder, with its own milk secretory tissue. This tissue consists of alveoli, ducts and connective tissue, which supports and protects the delicate secretory tissues (*see* diagram on page 28). The milk is synthesized by milk-component precursors being absorbed from the adjacent blood capillaries and converted into milk protein, lactose and fat in the secretory cells,

which are arranged as a single layer of cuboidal-shaped, epithelial cells on a basal membrane in the spherical structure called an alveolus. There are millions of alveoli which are the secretory units of the udder. The diameter of each alveolus is about 50–250μm. A cluster of alveoli separated from other clusters by fibrous connective tissue is known as a lobule and in turn a cluster of lobules is known as a lobe. The ducts draining the alveoli converge into larger intralobular ducts and then on to interlobular ducts, which drain into the gland cistern. The structure of this area is very similar to the structure of the lung. The milk is continuously synthesized in the alveolar area and stored in the alveoli, milk ducts and gland and teat cistern between milkings. 60–80 per cent of the milk is stored in the alveoli and small milk ducts, while the cistern contains only 20–40 per cent. However, there are relatively big differences between dairy cows when it comes to the cistern capacity. The amount of secretory tissue, or, in effect, the number of alveoli secretory cells, is the limiting factor for the milk producing capacity of the udder. It is a commonly held belief that a big udder is linked to a high milk production capacity. But this is not always true as a big udder might include a lot of connective and adipose tissue. Often these udders are referred to as having a lot of 'nature'. Udders with a high proportion of secretory tissue relative to connective tissue will appear quite flaccid after milking.

As milk accumulates in the alveoli between milking, the pressure on the epithelial lining causes the secretory cells to flatten under the back pressure and this, coupled with the collapse of the small capillaries reducing the supply of milk precursors, is thought to be part of the mechanism for switching off milk production.

Milking Frequency

A similar effect is seen with once-a-day milking, where yields can drop by 40 to 50 per cent, while omitting one milking a week, most popularly on a Sunday, would result in a drop in yield of 5 to 10 per cent. The converse effect of this is seen when cows show a yield increase

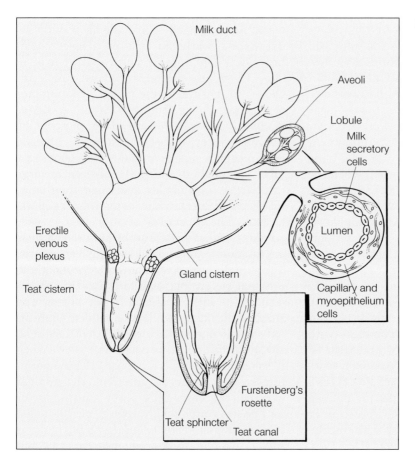

Microscopic udder anatomy.

of 10 to 15 per cent (heifers may be up to 15 to 20 per cent) with three times a day milking. This effect appears to be local to the quarter as cows with two quarters milked twice a day and two quarters milked four times a day will show an increase in yield only in the four-times-a-day milked quarters. If the effect were hormonal, say from oxytocin release into the blood, the effect of increased yield would be expected in all four quarters.

However, work at the Hannah Research Institute in Scotland, initially on goats, has shown that there is a second mechanism controlling milk production other than pressure feedback. An inhibitory protein was identified as providing a negative feedback on production. The increased removal of this inhibitory protein by four-times-a-day milking was compared to twice-a-day milking in the same cow by milking two quarters twice a day and two quarters four times a day. To prove that this was not a reduced back pressure effect, equal volumes of saline were infused back into the four-times-a-day milked quarters at two of the milkings and the yields still increased in the four-times-a-day milked quarters. After some months of four-times-a-day milking, the effect on those quarters was to increase the total amount of secretory tissue and not just to increase the secretory rate or yield. This effect is at the secretory tissue level, and so cows with large duct and cisternal capacity will tend to have higher yields because less of the inhibitory protein will be in contact with secretory tissue.

Milking Interval
The ideal interval is 12hr and 12hr with twice-a-day milking; this will give the highest yields.

However, many farms will have a shorter interval between the a.m. and the p.m. milking, as compared with the interval between the p.m. and the a.m. milking. Often this is 10hr and 14hr respectively, which, unless the cows are very high milkers, will not have an appreciable effect on lowering milk yields. Work from around the world has shown that even intervals of 16hr and 8hr will only cause a reduction of milk yield of 4 per cent and, although this was not deemed to be statistically significant, it is likely to become significant in high yielding cows.

MILK CONSTITUENTS

Milk Fat

Milk fat consists mainly of triglycerides, which are synthesized from glycerols and fatty acids. Long-chain fatty acids are absorbed from the blood and can be influenced by dietary fat. Dietary protected fats (fat which has been coated so it can bypass the rumen without being degraded) are included in dairy rations to improve milk butterfat. Short-chain fatty acids are synthesized in the mammary gland from components, such as acetate, which is absorbed from the rumen into the blood-stream. High-fibre diets, particularly long fibre, will increase the rumen production of acetate which will, in turn, raise milk butterfat. Stores of body fat can also influence the milk-fat levels.

Milk Protein

The main protein in milk is casein which is synthesized in the udder secretory cells from amino acids absorbed from the blood. Some albumen and immunoglobulins also move into the milk directly from the blood. Perhaps not intuitively, the effect of protein type and level in the diet has little impact on milk protein. However, the energy content of the diet significantly impacts milk protein to the extent that monitoring milk proteins at a bulk-milk-tank level, or more usefully by groups of cows at certain stages of lactation, can give a good insight into the energy adequacy of the diet.

Milk Lactose

Lactose is a disaccharide synthesized within the milk secretory cells from the combination of two sugars, glucose and galactose. In ruminants, glucose is produced in the liver from propionate, a volatile fatty acid and a product of rumen fermentation which is absorbed into the blood. Galactose is a derivative of glucose manufactured within the milk secretory cell.

Lactose is the major osmotically active milk constituent and alteration of lactose production has a marked influence on milk yield. For normal milk with a level of 4.5 to 5 per cent, lactose osmotic balance is reached. Lactose production acts as a regulator of the volume of milk produced by influencing the amount of water drawn into the secretory alveoli. Milk is isotonic with blood and, due to the presence of lactose, lower concentrations of sodium and chloride are needed in milk compared to levels in blood to compensate for the presence of lactose. Vitamins, minerals, salts and antibodies are transferred from the blood directly into the milk.

Dietary Influences

The diet fed to a dairy cow has a number of influences on both milk yield and milk constituents. There is a direct link with dietary energy intake and milk protein concentration (per cent protein), with low energy intakes resulting in depressed milk protein, while lack of sufficient fibre in the diet will depress milk fat concentrations (per cent butterfat). Milk yield itself is also influenced by the cow's energy intake by means of propionate production in the rumen, which, in turn, influences the glucose produced in the liver. The availability of glucose affects lactose production within the mammary gland, which, in turn, influences the milk yield by osmotic balancing within the gland.

DEFENCE MECHANISMS OF THE UDDER

The udder's defence against microbial invasion comprises a mix of non-specific and specific systems, including anatomical features which are covered in more detail elsewhere in the book and humoral (immune-based) and cellular mechanisms. Perhaps the most important defence mechanism of the mammary gland is the teat canal itself since this is the route of entry for most mastitis-causing micro-organisms. The teat canal acts as both a physical barrier, by impeding the entry of microbes, as well as being a source of various substances which have antimicrobial activity.

Non-specific Humoral Factors

*   *Lactoferrin* is discussed in detail in the section below on dry period.
*   *Lysosyme*
    An enzyme which can inhibit the growth of or destroy both Gram-positive and Gram-negative bacteria and can be derived either from blood or synthesized locally in the mammary gland; during inflammation it seems that leucocytes themselves appear to be the major source of lysosyme.
*   *Lactoperoxidase*
    The lactoperoxidase system, as with all peroxides (including peracetic acid-based disinfectants), operates by the generation of activated oxygen products which have a potent antibacterial action against most common udder pathogens *in vitro* at least (that is, in a laboratory situation, not in living tissue); however, this system appears to be inactivated by milk and hence has greater relevance in the dry period.
*   *Compliment*
    Compliment is known to play a role in the phagocytic killing of streptococcal species and the bactericidal effects of serum on *E.coli*.
*   *Cytokines*
    Cytokines are produced by immune cells and act as signalling proteins, providing local communication between the several cells of the immune system. These include interleukins, interferon and lymphokines, which are a type of cytokine released from lymphocytes. Cytokines can

encourage migration of neutrophils to an area of inflammation (calling in the soldiers), as well as speeding up the early involution of the mammary gland thus reducing the time when it is particularly susceptible to infection (possibly via the clearing up ability of neutrophils). In the future it may be possible to use cytokines as an alternative to antibiotic therapy for mastitis or as an adjuvant (helper) in any future vaccine use. Some workers have shown beneficial effects of both Interleukin-1 and Interferon gamma (IFN-g).

Specific Humoral Factors

*   *Immunoglobulins*
    Immunoglobulins are the most important specific humoral factors in the immune defence of the mammary gland. Immunoglobulin concentration in the mammary gland varies during the lactation cycle and is highest close to parturition. There is no immunoglobulin transfer to the calf *in utero* and so the early consumption of colostrum, which is high in IgG, IgA and IgM all at levels above that in the cow's blood, is essential for the acquisition of vital passive immunity for the newborn calf.

Cellular Defence

*   *Leucocytes*
    Leucocytes (white blood cells), and the small number of epithelial cells found in milk, are collectively known as somatic cells, alluded to in the term somatic cell count (SCC). The leucocytes in milk consist of lymphocytes, neutrophils and macrophages, which function in the generation of an effective immune response. Lymphocytes can be divided into two distinct subsets: T- and B-lymphocytes, which differ in function and protein products but tend to be involved in 'immune memory'. In the healthy gland, macrophages are the predominate cells and act as sentinels to invading mastitic pathogens. Once detected, macrophages release

chemoattractants, causing the recruitment and migration of large numbers of neutrophils and lymphocytes. However, this is a double-edged sword as, while neutrophils are phagocytosing and destroying the invading pathogens, they release chemicals which induce the swelling of secretory epithelium cytoplasm, the sloughing of secretory cells and decreased secretory activity. Resident and newly migrated macrophages help to reduce the damage to the epithelium by phagocytosing neutrophils that undergo programmed cell death through apoptosis. In spite of the considerable number of immune cells in the mammary gland, it has been suggested that the mammary gland is generally immunologically compromised when compared to the rest of the body. This may in part be due to the fact that the activity of all types of white cell (neutrophils, macrophages and lymphocytes) has been shown to be reduced within the mammary gland compared with these cells in blood.

- *Neutrophils*

Neutrophils are the most numerous white blood cells in the infected gland, accounting for up to 95 per cent of somatic cells:

The neutrophils' primary function is to phagocytose (to 'eat' and destroy) foreign material such as debris or bacteria, and again those in milk are less efficient at phagocytosis than those in blood;

Rapid deployment has been shown to be more important in limiting the severity of an acute *E.coli* mastitis than the absolute number of cells present before the infection;

Newly calved cows are slower to mobilize neutrophils after an infection than cows well into a lactation;

Neutrophils do not get recycled; the mammary gland is a terminal destination and some may be too mature (old) to be maximally effective, especially the first ones to arrive at the inflamed site;

With the massive recruitment of neutrophils once an infection has been established many arriving at the site of inflammation may be too young to be maximally effective;

Some of these less effective neutrophils may engulf the bacteria but may not kill them, thus offering them safe haven from the other immune defences the udder has. This may result in prolonging the bacterial infections;

Some neutrophils engorge themselves on milk fat and casein and tend to 'round up', becoming ineffective at ingesting bacteria;

Some bacteria, such as *Staphylococcus aureus*, appear to commonly resist intra cellular killing once internalized within the neutrophils, this allows them to continue living within the gland protected from the cow's defence mechanisms and able to reinfect the gland once the neutrophil dies and the bacteria are released. The normal lifespan of neutrophils in circulation is only a matter of a few hours but may be up to from five to seven days in tissue, and this is beyond the normal duration of intramammary antibiotic therapy. In this way the bacteria is also protected against the effects of treatment as most antibiotics used in mastitis treatment do not penetrate the neutrophil.

DRY PERIOD

The physiology of the mammary gland during the dry period differs markedly from that during lactation. There is a change from lactation (the wet milking period) through an involution period (a wet dry period) lasting a couple of weeks, to the true dry period (a dry dry period) which has a variable length dictated by the interval between dry off date and expected calving date. Then the udder regenerates again (a further wet dry period lasting a couple of weeks, often called the transition period) where the udder changes from a dry state to lactation.

These three phases described above are often referred to as:

1. active involution
2. steady state involution
3. redevelopment and colostrogenesis.

The susceptibility to mastitis, and thus the new infection rate, varies not only over the whole production cycle from lactation to dry period but also within both the lactation period and the dry period. During the dry period the most susceptible times are the two wet dry periods, just after drying off and just before calving.

Active Involution

(The early dry or first 'wet dry' period)
Active involution starts when the cow is milked for the last time in the current lactation. This can be as a result of drying off in a dairy cow or by weaning and removing the calf in a beef suckler cow. With either situation the cessation of milk removal will result in milk stasis. In the cow active involution takes about two weeks to complete and is a gradual process. It is a changeover phase of the mammary gland from the lactating to the non-lactating state. During this changeover phase a number of alterations occur in both the volume and the

composition of the mammary secretion. For a few days after drying off, milk continues to be produced. The udder will be visibly distended for up to one week, after which it will shrink rapidly to its dry state and the milk components, such as casein and milk fat, decline. The immunoglobulins (IgG, IgA and IgM) increase in concentration, but not as much as during colostrum formation just before calving.

Lactoferrin concentrations also increase considerably during the active involution phase. Lactoferrin is a globular multifunctional protein with antimicrobial activity (bactericidal, antiviral and fungicidal) and is part of the innate defence mechanism within the udder, particularly at the mucosal level. It is found not only in milk but in many other mucosal secretions, such as tears and saliva. Lactoferrin is an iron-binding protein and invading bacteria are forced to compete with lactoferrin for iron. Lactoferrin is also an antioxidant and limits the oxidative degeneration of cellular components that can occur during periods of tissue disruption, such as during inflammation and involution. Lactoferrin is also present in secondary

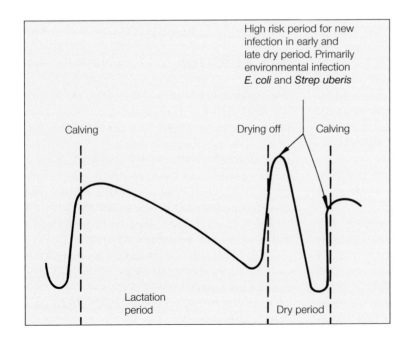

High risk period for new infection in early and late dry period. Primarily environmental infection *E. coli* and *Strep uberis*

Calving

Drying off

Calving

Lactation period

Dry period

Rate of new infections by stage of lactation.

granules of neutrophils and may play a role in the defence of the mammary gland by affecting the phagocytic activity of these cells.

Infections with environmentally-derived bacteria in the dry period are not uncommon, particularly in the two wet dry periods, the first two weeks and the last two weeks of the dry period. This is not surprising when you consider that once the cow has been dried off the risk of the spread of contagious pathogens within the milking parlour has effectively been eliminated. As a generalization, Gram-negative organisms (coliforms such as *E. coli*) are more common in the early dry period, while faecal streptococci such as *Streptococcus uberis* are more common in the late dry period. For coliform bacteria it is not just the levels of lactoferrin that are important but more the citrate:lactoferrin ratio. Citrate can bind or chelate iron and coliform bacteria can then use the citrate–iron complex for growth. During early involution citrate concentration declines and, despite the lactoferrin concentration increasing, the availability of iron is sufficient so that the mammary gland does not have a reduced succeptibilty to coliform infection, unlike later in the dry period.

The cellular make-up of the secretions from the involuting mammary gland varies from that of the lactating gland. The majority of cells are white blood cells, or leucocytes, with a few shedding epithelial cells. The total leucocyte concentration in mammary secretions increases rapidly in early involution, although the population will change in type over time. Phagocytic leucocytes, or neutrophils, predominate for the first three to seven days after drying off. However, if the quarter is also infected they will have been present throughout the early stages of infection, as evidenced by a raised SCC. After about a week, the population has more macrophages present and these are also phagocytic. Many are filled with ingested fat droplets and other debris. They play an important role in removing large quantities of fat and cellular debris, including dead neutrophils. There is always a proportion of lymphocytes present and these

tend to mirror the increase in macrophage population becoming the predominant cell type in the mid dry dry period.

The following factors increase the risk of a new intramammary infection during the early dry period:

- cessation of milking
  - milk is no longer intermittently removed by milking
  - no flushing out of bacteria
  - milk accumulates in the udder after initial drying off
  - increased intramammary pressure compromises the streak canal, resulting in leakage of milk from the teats
  - teat-end disinfection is stopped
  - bacteria can grow well in milk
- changes in udder environment
  - leucocytes become engorged by ingesting milk fat, casein and debris
  - protective lactoferrin and immunoglobulin concentrations are slow to rise
  - citrate:lactoferrin ratio is high favouring Gram-negative infections.

The use of antibiotic dry cow therapy (DCT), administered at drying off, is a useful tool to help eliminate existing infections, as well as affording some protection against new infections while the product is active. The use of teat seals, either in the form of external (Dry Flex, DeLaval) or internal (Orbeseal, Pfizer Animal Health) can also help in reducing new infections in this early dry period. *See* the section on dry cow therapy, Chapter 7.

Steady State Involution
(The mid dry or 'dry dry' period)
he length of the steady state involution dry period depends on the total length of the dry period; if active involution takes about two weeks to complete in the dairy cow and the redevelopment stage takes about two weeks, then that accounts for four weeks, leaving from two to four weeks of steady state involution, if the total dry period is the traditional six to eight weeks (or often quoted as forty-five to

sixty days). Cows with shorter dry periods will have mammary tissue undergoing active involution and beginning the redevelopment phase concurrently. This may contribute to a decline in the optimal milk yield in the next lactation. However, other factors (metabolic and management factors) also contributed to the original traditional requirement for the forty-five to sixty days dry period, as, in fact, they do to the more recent moves to shorter dry periods.

New intramammary infection rates are generally low during the steady state phase period. This is the period of greatest resistance to intramammary infection; if an infection does occur in the steady state dry period it is often eliminated spontaneously. Additionally, if an infection exists prior to drying off this is the period where spontaneous recovery is most likely to occur. Shorter dry periods will shorten this steady state and may reduce self-cure of existing intramammary infections.

Factors reducing the risk of a new intramammary infection during the mid dry period:

- the udder has adapted to a steady state of involution
  - very little fluid volume in the udder
  - a proportion of teats have become sealed reducing the chance of leakage
- favourable changes in udder environment
  - the udder environment is less conducive to bacterial growth
  - little milk fat, casein or debris left and so leucocytes are more effective
  - lactoferrin and immunoglobulin concentration are high
  - citrate:lactoferrin ratio is lowered.

Redevelopment and Colostrogenesis
(The late dry or second 'wet dry' period)
This phase of the dry period describes the transition from non-lactating to lactating status and is often referred to as the transition period. There is no predetermined time or trigger for this process to start, but it is generally seen as the udder starts to 'spring' in the two weeks leading up to calving. Obvious visible signs of udder regeneration start ten to fourteen days before the impending parturition and are very obvious from three to five days before calving. The reason for the late dry period being a higher risk for intramammary infection, like the early dry period, is because the changes in the udder environment are similar but in the opposite direction:

- milk accumulates in the udder as calving approaches
  - increased intramammary pressure compromises streak canal integrity and can result in leakage of milk from the teats
  - teat-end disinfection may be performed before calving but often is not initiated until after calving
  - bacteria can grow well in milk
- changes in udder environment
  - leucocytes are faced with increasing milk fat, and casein again
  - lactoferrin has declined significantly as calving approaches
  - citrate:lactoferrin ratio is high, favouring Gram-negative infections again
  - unlike lactoferrin, immunoglobulin (antibody) levels increase significantly and are being actively accumulated in the colostrums.

As this period of increased risk approaches, dry cow therapy has often ceased to be active. The limited time of action in the dry period is to ensure that milk from cows once calved have milk antibiotic residues below the maximum residue limit (MRL) set by the EU for UK milk production. It is possible to improve the protection against new intramammary infections in the late dry period by the use of teat seals, either in the form of external (Dry Flex; De Laval) or internal (Orbeseal, Pfizer Animal Health). (*See* the section on dry cow therapy, Chapter 7.)

CHAPTER THREE

Mastitis: What Causes It and How to Control It

MASTITIS: KNOW YOUR ENEMY

Origins of Mastitis Infections

Overt clinical mastitis cases can be the result of a new infection in a previously uninfected quarter or of the fulmination of an existing sub-clinical infection. An existing sub-clinical infection may also be the result of a new infection in a previously uninfected quarter which remains a 'silent' infection and can be detected only by a test procedure such as SCC or bacteriology. New mastitis infections, which, by definition, can occur only in previously uninfected quarters, may originate from either another infected quarter in the same cow, or in another cow (contagious spread) or from sources other than infected quarters, such as faecal contamination (environmental spread).

Prevalence and Incidence

Prevalence
Prevalence is the proportion of a population having a disease at a given time.
Incidence
Incidence is the number of cases of disease in a given time period; incidence is usually expressed for a given population, for example, cases per hundred cows per year.

It is possible for a herd to have a high prevalence and a low incidence of mastitis and vice versa. This has significance when assessing a herd for mastitis status. Mastitis records will, if accurate, give an indication of mastitis incidence, whereas BMSCC might give a better indication of prevalence.

Compare two herds: one has a BMSCC of 350,000 cells/ml and a mastitis incidence of twenty cases per hundred cows per year. The other has a BMSCC of <100,000 cells/ml and a mastitis incidence of 180 cases per hundred cows per year. Which herd would you like to be in?

Establishment of Infection

The inherent virulence of a bacterial species is often associated with its ability to adhere to mammary epithelium and remain in the gland during lactation, despite the udder being effectively but periodically flushed by the milking process. *Streptococcus agalactiae* and *Staphylococcus aureus* adhere well, *E. coli* does not adhere well but multiplies rapidly so the population survives the flushing process. Bacteria initially affect tissues lining the large milking collecting ducts and cisterns. They enter small ducts and alveolar areas of the gland by multiplication and via milk currents. Some bacteria produce toxins and irritants that cause swelling and death of alveoli. This results in the release of substances that increase blood-vessel permeability and attract neutrophils to the affected area.

PREDISPOSING FACTORS

Mastitis, like many infections, is a balance, or perhaps more an imbalance, between the

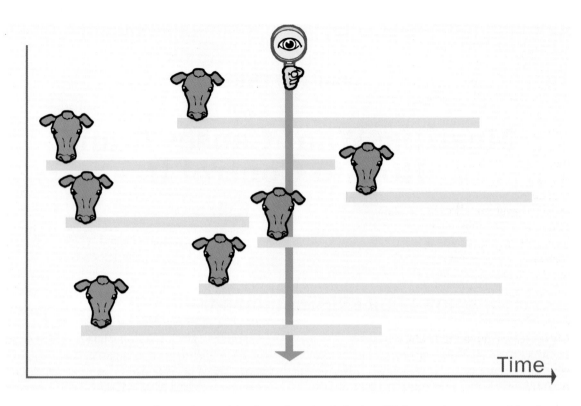

Comparison of incidence and prevalence with a long duration infection. High prevalence even with a low new infection rate, e.g. Staphylococcus aureus.

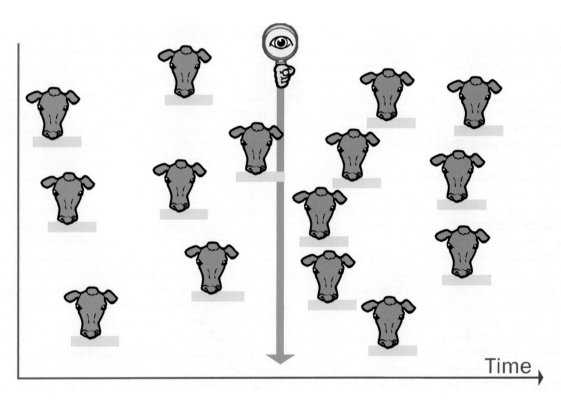

Comparison of incidence and prevalence with a short duration infection. Low prevalence even with a high new infection rate, e.g. E. coli.

pathogen (the bug), the host (the cow) and the environment (the surroundings). An infection of the mammary gland will occur when a population of pathogenic bacteria becomes established. The imbalance can be a high enough bacterial challenge or a sufficiently virulent strain to overcome a cow with a normal immune system or a cow with a compromised immune system, allowing an infection to establish from a challenge a normal cow would eliminate. In a similar way, predisposing factors tend to either compromise the cow's defence mechanisms or deliver high infective doses of pathogenic bacteria.

Cow Factors

Cow factors have the potential to have both positive and negative effects on a cow's susceptibility to mastitis. Historically, selective breeding in dairy cattle has been based on phenotype, the outward physical characteristics, that make a first class dairy cow. Selection is based on the traits that are thought to ensure longevity. These will include body conformation (specifically body shape and size, which will relate to general wellbeing and, more specifically, appetite capacity), with good legs and feet (which will relate to mobility and lack of a predisposition to lameness) and udder conformation, with again emphasis on size and shape with good udder attachment and teat shape and positioning. These physical characteristics will be heritable to an extent and dairy farmers have long recognized family lines having both advantageous and, in some cases, deleterious traits and have selectively bred replacement cattle accordingly. This type of selection is based on the female line, by farmers recognizing cows within their herd having desirable traits. The selection of bulls to use on these cows has to be based on data from daughters of the bull. This takes time to accumulate and is to a certain extent complicated by the need to compensate for the myriad of cows used to breed the daughters to get the data. The beneficial trait from either a cow or a bull will, in effect, be diluted as each supplies only half the genetic material for the offspring.

Heritability helps to explain the degree to which genes control expression of a trait, for example, resistance to clinical mastitis. Heritability is a measure of the degree (0 to 1) to which offspring resemble their parents for a specific trait. Heritability measures the strength of the relationship between performance, say, mastitis rate in a cow (phenotype) and breeding value, and the likely reduction in mastitis rate passed on to the offspring (genotype) of an individual animal. Heritability of production traits such as milk yield (0.3) or milk protein content (0.5) are high, but still more effect comes from non-genetic influences such as nutrition, 'breeding up' to Holstein Friesian from British Friesian or environmental management, and so selective breeding will make relatively slow progress.

The heritability of both the SCC level and resistance to clinical mastitis are often quoted as between 0.1 and 0.2, with SCC generally having the higher heritability, which makes progress on udder health by genetic selection a matter of decades of breeding rather than years. Positive values to improve traits for udder health (SCC or clinical mastitis) tend to have an association with a negative effect on yield. Careful bull selection is needed to improve udder health without adversely affecting yield. Available and accurate clinical mastitis data are very sparse in the dairy industry the world over, unlike SCC data which are both accurate and available. Research work has shown that daughters of sires that transmit the lowest SCC score had the lowest incidence of clinical mastitis and the fewest clinical episodes during first and second lactations, making SCC a good proxy measure for genetic selection for udder health. Recent and on-going work in Holland has shown that if one uses the SCC data in a smart way by looking at the number and duration of peaks of SCC >150 as well as SCC in early lactation, rather than simple SCC averages for the whole lactation – which can be very misleading – the accuracy of estimated breeding values may be significantly improved. In fact, this work shows that the need for clinical mastitis data (which are rarely complete or accurate), although still essential for accurate mastitis breeding value for sires, can be some-what mitigated by this smarter use of SCC data. This means that breeding values can be estimated more accurately and more quickly (without waiting for clinical data), with the result that good and less good sires can be better distinguished. However, the Dutch research workers will continue to look at the evaluation of clinical data where it is available in sentinel herds. This research work, in common with that of other workers from around the world, concluded that the best parameters for deter-mining an udder health index were SCC (low), fore udder attachment (tight), front teat place-ment (narrow), teat length (short), udder depth (shallow) and milking speed (optimal is mid speed). Most countries use the same param-eters, although milking speed is not as widely recognized or used and there may well be dif-ferences between the availability of data, aims and possible effects of AMS (robot) milking and conventional parlours.

Non-specific disease interactions such as concurrent disease, particularly periparturi-ent disease, such as milk fever, metritis and abomasal disorders, will increase mastitis sus-ceptibility as well as more specific interactions, such as bovine virus diarrhoea (BVD) which can cause generalized immunosuppresion.

Pathogen Factors

The details of the specific pathogens causing mastitis, listed under the Specific Causes of Mastitis section later in the chapter, indicate the influence pathogen type has on the vari-ability in mastitis. Pathogens have to invade and multiply to survive being flushed out by milking or being destroyed by the cow's defence mechanisms.

Milking Machine Factors

The milking parlour can have a considerable influence on new infection rates with both con-tagious pathogens and environmental patho-gens. The mechanism for the spread of a con-tagious pathogen within the parlour is perhaps more obvious, with the fomite spread that can occur via infected milk within the liner causing a new infection in the next six to eight cows milked after an infected cow has been milked. Fomite spread within the parlour can also occur via the milker's hands or the multi-use cloths or towels. The milking machine can also influence new infection rates with environmental infec-tions. The milking machine can be the final pathway by which the bacteria present on the teat skin before milking or in the milk during milking can be driven in through the streak canal by retrograde flow of milk. The poten-tial for this retrograde flow will be increased in poorly maintained milking machines or ones with inadequate vacuum reserves.

However, even in an up-to-date, well main-tained parlour there is still a potential for the retrograde flow of milk and this will be most likely to occur when there are vacuum fluctua-tions in the liner, particularly at the teat end. These vacuum fluctuations are most common when milk flow rates are either very high at peak flow or low at the beginning or the end of the milking of each cow, or if air leaks occur as liner slips. At very high peak flow rates the capacity of the milking machine to remove milk efficiently from the cluster, and thus away from the teat end, can be overcome and 'flood-ing' can occur, bathing the teats in potentially infected milk. At the beginning or at the end of the milking of each cow, when milk flow rates are low, effects on vacuum stability can result in the retrograde flow of milk such that 'impacts' occur where the milk can be force-fully driven on to the teat end. Both 'flooding' and 'impacts' can significantly increase the risk of infection penetrating the streak canal. *See* the diagram on page 81, Chapter 4.

A well maintained, clean modern milking machine working to the latest British Standards (BS ISO 6690, 5707 and 5545) required by the Assured Dairy Farms (ADF) formerly the National Dairy Farm Assured Scheme (NDFAS) is essential to produce high quality milk for the current market place.

Environmental Factors

The importance of the environment encom-passes many aspects that impinge on the likelihood of an intramammary infection occurring, including the most obvious association with the terms environment and environmental mastitis, and that is hygiene. However, there are a number of other influences the environment will have on mastitis infection rates, including the ambient temperature, humidity, space availability in terms of comfort (which is effectively straw yard stocking density or number of cubicles available) and lying times (time spent lying down). When a cow is lying down, blood flow to the udder increases by 30 per cent. Therefore the clear message from this for dairy farmers is that if a cow is not eating, drinking or being milked, she should be lying down. As a general guide, only 10 per cent of cows should be standing up at 10.00pm.

Human Factors

The job of a dairy stockperson is highly skilled and their ability will influence farm mastitis rates quite dramatically. This can be a real effect in terms of the actual number of mastitis cases occurring related to their diligence and husbandry skills. However, as the diagnosis is made by the stockperson the treatment rate can be influenced by the individual's approach to treatment in mild cases. As some very mild cases will self-cure, some milkers will wait 12hr (for the next milking) to see whether the case is real and needs treating, while others will treat much more readily. In the instance of a very mild coliform case that has self-cured but was treated, the cure will be attributed to the treatment, but perhaps more significantly, the case will be recorded in the farm mastitis rate. With the farm that waits 12hr and the case is seen to self-cure there will be no treatment record, which will effectively reduce the mastitis rate. As a consequence, the mastitis rate is determined by the dairy stockperson, in terms of both true infection rate and the treatment rate (recorded cases).

The herd size or, more significantly, the stockperson to cow ratio, will also have a significant effect on the ability of even the most skilled worker to manage the herd effectively and this will certainly apply to mastitis control.

Nutritional Factors

Some would say that nutrition underpins all disease processes, and it is true to say that cows in significant negative energy balance (NEB), where nutritional demands outstrip the supply of nutrients from the diet, will be susceptible to a whole range of metabolic diseases and more prone to infectious diseases, of which mastitis is only one. Any nutritional inadequacies will result in generalized and non-specific negative effects on the immune system.

More specific nutritional factors, such as mineral deficiencies, can have a role. Work particularly from the USA has implicated selenium/vitamin E deficiency as being associated with elevated SCC and possibly increased clinical mastitis rates. Selenium (Se) and vitamin E are integral components of the antioxidant defence of tissues and cells, and a known consequence of vitamin E and selenium deficiency is impaired white blood cell activity in terms of both the cells' production in response to an infectious challenge and their killing ability.

Nutrition can also influence mastitis rates in an indirect fashion by affecting faecal consistency. A well formulated diet, creating a

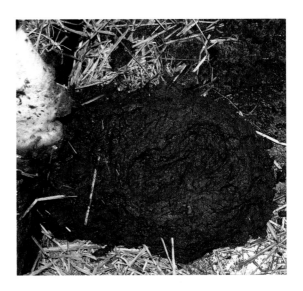

Good faecal consistency reduces contamination of the udder. Note the 'rosebud' depression in the cow pat.

firm dung pat, will greatly reduce the faecal contamination of the teat ends and so help to reduce environmental humidity and the risk of environmental mastitis. The ideal cow pat should be well formed, stand up a couple of centimetres and have an indent the size of a rosebud formed by the last faecal output.

Categorization of Mastitis

What Types Are There?

Mastitis can be subdivided into categories based on the effect it has on the udder and the cow, the type of pathogen or the origin of the pathogen that caused it. Further categorization in more broad terms is often used to distinguish clinical mastitis, where changes to the milk are detectable to the naked eye (clots or flakes) and sub-clinical mastitis, where detection relies on a test procedure as milk changes are not visible to the naked eye. Tests used to detect sub-clinical mastitis are based either on a direct approach, such as bacteriological culture to identify the causal bacteria or an indirect approach based on a measure of either the inflammatory response within the udder, or the detection of changes in the milk composition. Measurement of SCC is perhaps the most common example of an indirect method of indicating inflammation and can be measured either quantitatively by a commercial company (such as NMR – National Milk Records, or CIS – Cattle Information Service) or semi-quantitatively by a rapid mastitis test, such as the California Milk Test (CMT). Bacteriological culture would then often be used to identify the cause once the infected quarters had been identified by using SCC estimation.

Electroconductivity can also be used as an indirect measure to indicate a degree of compositional changes in the milk and is available automatically at each milking in some modern parlours and in particular in Automatic Milking Systems (AMS or robotic milking). Other markers for mastitis which can be useful are inflammatory proteins and chemical mediators, but these are used more in research as they are not immediate and measurement tends to be more costly. Diagnostic methods are covered in more detail in Chapter 6.

Presentation

Clinical

Per-acute This is most commonly seen as a rapid onset of severe inflammation of the udder, resulting in a hot, swollen quarter with an abnormal secretion which may often be watery and accompanied by a severely systemically ill cow, which in some cases may be fatal. The systemic illness often appears before changes are seen in the milk or udder. Per-acute mastitis can lead to the cessation of milk production (agalactiae). The systemic illness is often due to septicaemia or toxaemia, resulting in a rapid pulse, fever, depression, decreased rumen motility, loss of appetite and scouring (diarrhoea). The progression of this condition may result in dehydration, recumbency and end in the death of the cow.

Acute Acute mastitis is most often seen as a sudden onset of moderate to severe inflammation of the udder with a decrease in milk production and sometimes watery milk but more often clots. Systemic signs are similar to those of the per-acute form but less severe.

Subacute Mastitis Sub-acute mastitis is most frequently seen as a mild inflammation, often with no visible changes in the udder. There will often be small flakes or clots in the milk, which may have an off-colour. There are no systemic signs of illness.

Chronic A long-term and frequently recurring condition is said to be chronic (from the Greek *chronos*). Chronic mastitis may persist in a sub-clinical form for months or even years with occasional clinical flare-ups. Sometimes these repeat clinical cases can lead to permanent udder damage, resulting in scarring and induration which can result in micro-abscessation and the walling off of infection. The udder can become noticeably uneven and hard; these changes are irreversible and will often result in the need to cull the cow.

Sub-clinical

Sub-clinical mastitis is the most common form. It is fifteen to forty times more common than clinical mastitis. There is no gross inflammation of the udder and no gross changes in the milk. There is decreased production and lowered milk quality.

TYPES OF PATHOGEN

Major

Major mastitis pathogens are generally the bacteria commonly associated with clinical mastitis. These are generally accepted to be *Streptococcus agalactiae*, *Staphylococcus aureus*, *Streptococcus uberis*, *Streptococcus dysgalactiae*, coliforms (such as *E. coli*, *Klebsiella* spp., *Enterobacter* spp. and *Citrobacter* spp.) and *Pseudomonas* spp. Other pathogens include mycoplasmas (which are not common in the United Kingdom as a cause of mastitis but are significant in the USA, Canada, Israel, Australia, New Zealand and several countries in Europe), protatheca and yeasts such as candida.

Minor

These bacteria are often viewed as normal commensals of the mammary gland and can be considered as part of the normal natural bacterial flora of the udder. However, they have a complex interaction with the udder and can be involved in SCC elevation. The most common minor pathogens are coagulase-negative *Staphylococci* and coryneform bacteria such as *Corynebacterium bovis*. These bacteria have an ability to produce natural antibacterial substances which may offer protection from intramammary infection by major pathogens and are also considered to have a beneficial effect by competitive inhibition.

ORIGINS OF INFECTION

Environmental

Environmental mastitis denotes mastitis that spreads from the environment to the cow. The incidence of environmental mastitis can often increase as the incidence of contagious mastitis decreases or at least becomes proportionately more important. The principal habitat of bacteria causing environmental mastitis is, unsurprisingly, the environment (faeces, soil, bedding or water). The disease is often taken to be the result of faecal contamination, usually the most significant source with coliform bacteria, such as *E. coli*; however, there are also 'true' environmental bacteria where the cow's environment is the source, such as *Pseudomonas*. Infection can occur from contact of the teats at milking time or between milkings. The major organisms causing environmental mastitis include the Gram-negative coliform bacteria such as *E. coli* or *Klebsiella*, the environmental streptococcal species such as *Streptococcus uberis*, and *Pseudomonas* species, but other organisms found in the cow's environment can cause mastitis too.

Contagious

Contagious mastitis denotes mastitis that spreads from cow to cow. The principal habitat of bacteria causing contagious mastitis is either on or in infected mammary glands and sometimes in infected teat lesions. Contagious bacteria tend to survive less well outside the infected cows, needing to have relatively close direct contact for spread or occasionally indirect contact by a fomite. Chronic or sub-clinical mastitis is most commonly associated with bacteria which cause contagious mastitis. The infection is transmitted by milk-contaminated fomites at milking, by multi-use udder cloths, by the milker's hands, and by the milking machine. The major organisms causing contagious mastitis are *Streptococcus agalactiae*, *Staphylococcus aureus* and *Mycoplasma*.

The distinction between environmental and contagious mastitis, although convenient for a generalized approach, does not always withstand more detailed scrutiny for certain pathogens. There are examples of both contagious pathogens behaving in an environmental fashion and environmental pathogens behaving in a contagious fashion. Research has shown that *Staphylococcus aureus* can be isolated from bedding samples apparently free living without close contact with skin or the udder, and other work has shown it to be potentially transmitted by flies. On the other hand, research using strain typing has shown that *Streptococcus uberis* can cause persistent chronic infections which result in increased SCC and a potential to spread in a contagious manner.

SPECIFIC CAUSES OF MASTITIS

Despite the fact that most bovine mastitis is caused almost exclusively by bacteria and that there are many potential pathogens, the vast majority of cases are caused by just a few bacterial types. This does make laboratory identification of causal pathogens easier than if the causal agents were many and varied.

For practical purposes, the most common causes of mastitis can be counted on one hand, although there are clearly many other and less common causes, and some of the groups, in particular the Gram-negative bacilli, can be subdivided. However, *Streptococcus agalactiae*, *Staphylococcus aureus*, *Streptococcus uberis*, *Streptococcus dysgalactiae* and *E. coli* would account for the vast majority of cases.

Staphylococcus aureus
Staphylococcus aureus remains a significant cause of both clinical and sub-clinical mastitis in cattle, which is in no small part due to the fact that the elimination of this infection from an infected lactating mammary gland can be difficult. The fact that the dairy industry has not eradicated *Streptococcus agalactiae* from the global dairy herd is more to do with the lack of determination to apply control measures and herd biosecurity rigorously rather than its not being a realistic goal. However, the goal of *Staphylococcus aureus* eradication from an individual herd, let alone the national or global herd, is not a realistic one as the bacterium is not an obligate udder pathogen and can survive in the cow environment. It is not as closely or even exclusively associated with

Key Points

- Contagious – spreads from cow to cow
- Cattle are the most common source of infection
- Sub-clinical infection is common
- Clinical cases can be difficult to treat, particularly when well established
- Causes long-term damage to the udder
- Risk factors – purchase of infected cattle
- Cannot effectively or practically be eradicated from a herd
- Identify significantly infected herds by bulk milk culture or cows with high SCCs
- Often a stealth bug, with variable increases in SCC and intermittent bacterial excretion
- Shows significant strain variation, resulting in differences in ease of successful treatment, degree of damage to the udder and elevation of SCC
- Can originate from sources other than cows, such as milkers' hands, fomites and flies
- Control – five-point plan, good milking routine, wearing gloves and vigilant use of antibiotic for all clinical cases, and all cows at drying off coupled, with culling of persistently infected cows.

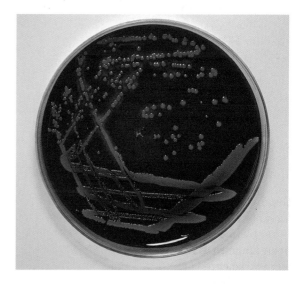

Staphylococcus aureus cultured on blood agar.

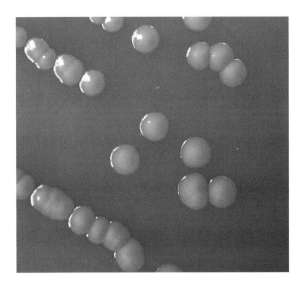

Golden yellow oil-drop colonies typical of Staphylococcus aureus.

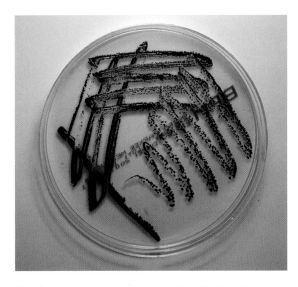

Staphylococcus aureus cultured on Baird Parker, a selective medium.

Laboratory Characteristics

- Grows on blood agar and selective media such as Baird Parker
- 3–4mm oil-drop colonies
- Colonies golden yellow on blood agar and generally haemolytic
- Gram-positive cocci; *see* photo on page 154, Chapter 6
- Catalase-positive; *see* photo on page 154, Chapter 6
- Coagulase-positive, although some strains can be coagulase-negative; this may be a true lack of coagulase activity in some strains or may be due to the sensitivity of the coagulase test being employed; *see* photo on page 155, Chapter 6.

the cow's udder and skin as *Streptococcus agalactiae* but is still very much a bacterium that is happy in and around the cow. Attempts have been made to eradicate *Staphylococcus aureus* from a selected group of high health status dairy herds and run them as *Staphylococcus aureus-* free herds. However, the sources of *Staphylococcus aureus* other than from infected cows is sufficient to make this goal unattainable. Unlike *Streptococcus agalactiae* where biosecurity based on the avoidance of purchasing infected cattle will suffice, merely avoiding purchasing *Staphylococcus aureus*-infected cattle into a *Staphylococcus aureus*-free herd will not guarantee avoiding the reintroduction of *Staphylococcus aureus* into the herd. *Staphylococcus aureus* infections are chiefly spread at milking time via fomites such as the cluster and the milker's hands. Although individual infected quarters generally have an elevated cell count, *Staphylococcus aureus* is often seen as a stealth bug and, in the early stages, can be present in quarters without causing a large inflammatory response in terms of SCC elevation and tissue changes. However, although uncommon, *Staphylococcus aureus* cases can develop into a severe gangrenous mastitis, resulting in the sloughing of the affected quarter. New infections in the initial stages after invasion of the mammary gland can, if detected, often be treated successfully. As they become more chronic they tend to cause a greater inflammatory response, resulting in permanent changes to the secretory tissue often becoming walled off with scar tissue within the udder, which inevitably results in poorer responses

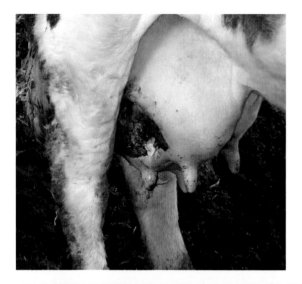

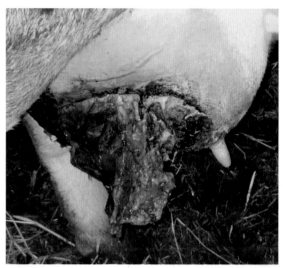

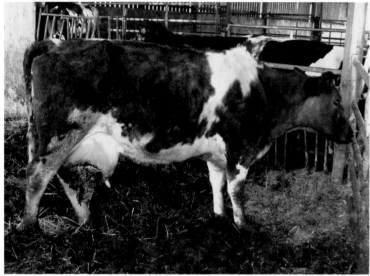

Gangrenous mastitis resulting in sloughing of the affected quarter.

to treatment. The inflammatory response seen in the infected gland will vary with time. Variation will be seen over a time period in terms of fluctuating SCCs and intermittent excretion, as well as with time in terms of the increasing pathology seen in chronic infections. These more chronic changes can result in permanent changes to the udder which can be detected both by palpating and on occasions by visual examination. The detection of a hard, lumpy, indurated udder is a good indicator that the cow has suffered repeated bouts of infection and inflammation and may well be a carrier cow with a chronic long-term infection and an elevated SCC. Cows with these udder changes are likely to pose a risk to the rest of the herd and the udder changes make it highly unlikely that they can be cured or will be capable of producing low SCC milk. The intermittent excretion in the milk exhibited by some cows infected with *Staphylococcus aureus* may be for a number of reasons. One reason may be that *Staphylococcus aureus* can resist the killing effects of neutrophils

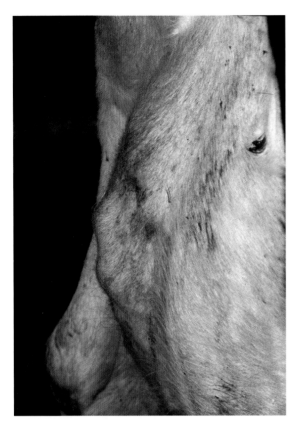

Indurated, hard, knobbly udder typical of chronic Staphylococcus aureus infection.

once they are phagocytosed (or 'eaten'), which means that not only do they effectively hide from the immune system for that time, but they can also reinfect the udder when they are released back into it when the neutrophils die. This may be a reflection or even cause of the fluctuating cell counts seen with quarters infected with *Staphylococcus aureus*.

It can be surmised that, as the exposure of the mammary immune system to an infectious agent will be one of the reasons for a rise in SCC, the fact that *Staphylococcus aureus* can effectively hide by both becoming walled off and/or surviving phagocytosis, the presentation of the bacteria to the immune system will be variable. This can result in cyclical fluctuations in SCC: the bacteria are killed by the cow's immune system thus reducing the challenge that was originally driving up the SCCs and, as a consequence, the SCC will gradually drop as the immune system is no longer seeing a huge bacterial challenge, which then allows any surviving bacteria to start to multiply again, triggering a rise in SCC again. The intermittent excretion in milk exhibited by *Staphylococcus aureus* and its ability to survive within neutrophils has a significant impact on the sensitivity of bacteriological culture as a

Variation in *Staphylococcus aureus* excretion and quarter SCC over time

Date	Bacteria	cfu	¼ Cell count	Possible scenario
23/06/97	*C+Staph*	6	987	SCC response to high number of cfus
30/06/97	*C+Staph*	100	661	
29/07/97	No growth		754	SCC activity causes reduction in cfu excretion and SCC drops
05/08/97	*C+Staph*	20	21	
13/08/97	*C+Staph*	100	5531	Allowing bacterial multiplication which causes SCC to rise again
02/10/97	*C+Staph*	100	167	Unclear scenario between cfu and SCC

Sampling this cow on 29/7/97 would not have yielded *Staphylococcus aureus* – the likely causal bacteria.
Source: Biggs, 1997, unpublished.

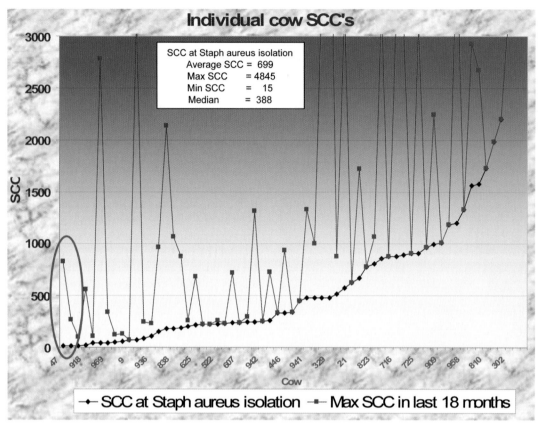

Variation in SCC in Staphylococcus aureus-infected cows. The two cows with SCC of 15 at isolation have max SCCs of 269 and 826.

method of diagnosis of *Staphylococcus aureus* intramammary infection. With clinical cases of *Staphylococcus aureus* the numbers of bacteria shed in the milk are usually high and continuous and bacteriological diagnosis is generally easy. However, with sub-clinical cases, where inflammatory changes are less marked and bacterial excretion more variable, false negative results are not uncommon. Sensitivity of bacterial culture as a mean of diagnosis for *Staphylococcus aureus* can be improved by a combination of pre-culture processing and repeat sampling. Repeat sampling will improve the sensitivity of detection by overcoming intermittent excretion, and it has been suggested that, while a single sample has an approximately 75 per cent sensitivity, two samples increase this to 94 per cent sensitivity, and three samples may

achieve 98 per cent sensitivity. The freezing of samples prior to culture will also improve *Staphylococcus aureus* detection rates as a result of the release of bacteria from within neutrophils. The expansion of ice crystals as they form when milk is frozen will cause the rupturing of cells within the milk, releasing intracellular *Staphylococcus aureus* from within neutrophils and making them available for culture. Despite these techniques, *Staphylococcus aureus* detection even in known infected quarters can be difficult and may be improved further by the use of selective media, such as Baird Parker. *See* ISQT in Chapter 6.

Improving detection rates is essential in *Staphylococcus aureus* control as identifying both individual infected cows and determining herd prevalence are critical in formulating a *Staphylococcus aureus* control programme. There are no prizes for keeping a herd *Staphylococcus aureus*-free nor is there extra income based on milk price. However, an achievable and desirable target would be to keep *Staphylococcus aureus* at a level where there is no discernible economic impact either by clinical disease or milk quality. A common approach to mastitis control in general, which would apply equally well to *Staphylococcus aureus* control, would be monitoring of bulk samples, say, on a quarterly basis, combined

Staphylococcus aureus risk factors and control measures

Risk factors	Control measures
Purchasing infected cows	Keep a closed herd. Biosecurity
Inadequate post-milking teat disinfection (partial teat coverage, wrong dilution, part year teat dipping, poor quality dip)	Adequate post-milking dipping year round
Hand stripping, shared udodercloths and not wearing gloves	Good hygiene at teat preparation
Cow to cow transmission via cluster	Separate cluster for mastitic cows. Milk infected cows last (clinical and/or subclinical). Identify problem cows early. Manual or automatic cluster disinfection
Poor diagnosis of clinical cases	Improve diagnosis of clinical mastitis, by sampling
Inadequate treatment and recording of clinical cases. (Tube usage and type, records and use of records)	Improve treatment success by selecting appropriate therapy regimes and treatment
Faulty parlour function or design	Check for small claw pieces, vacuum fluctuations within the claw or claw piece flooding
Poor maintenance of the parlour. Inadequate plant cleaning	Ensure a policy is in place for regular servicing and rubberware replacement. Look at cleaning regimes
Damaged teat orifice post-milking	Check for pulsator malfunction, vacuum levels, over-milking, excessive use of lime in cubicles
Partial dry cow therapy (only some cows treated, poor technique, milk run out after tubing, inadequate length of treatment)	Ensure all cows are treated with DCT. Match activity of tube to length of dry period. Ensure clean infusion technique is used
Inconsistent culling policy (infected cows not culled, old cows with high cell counts present in herd)	Identify high cell count cows to be culled via reliable records. Include repeat offenders and older cows

with the sampling of CMT positive quarters from high SCC cows identified by routine composite cow SCC samples through monthly milk recording. Depending on the current and historic BMSCC, action would be taken on either positive *Staphylococcus aureus* culture in bulk milk or at an individual cow level. A positive *Staphylococcus aureus* culture from a bulk milk sample would warrant further investigation at a cow level, especially if BMSCC was at or close to a level where financial penalties would be incurred. Once an individual cow is identified as being infected with *Staphylococcus aureus* there is often little chance of successful treatment. The best chance of a cure is during the dry period and in younger cows with single quarters infected and no previous history of either clinical episodes or elevated SCC. However, work in Israel showed that the treatment of even established *Staphylococcus aureus* infections can be successful if treated with extended therapy, in this case twenty-one tubes were used. This work was not, as the author said, to encourage the dairy industry to treat with such long courses of antibiotic but to show what could be achieved. Other treatment protocols can improve cure rates, such as combination therapy (injection plus intramammary tubes) or pulse therapy (sequential repeated datasheet treatment including the milk withhold – resulting in a pulsed or on/off treatment often used with three pulses). There is, as with many infectious agents, a degree of *Staphylococcus aureus* strain variation which is reflected in the severity, persistence and contagiousness of the disease exhibited in an infected udder. Although strain typing is not commercially available, various fingerprinting techniques have been used to identify common strains within herds or persistent strains within cows. Besides these more subtle fingerprinting differences, there are more fundamental differences between strains, for example, where certain strains are known to produce penicillinase, an enzyme which destroys some penicillin-based antibiotics. Penicillinase production has been linked with

virulence, although this may have more relevance in the human field.

The outcome of treatment of a *Staphylococcus aureus*-infected gland may well be predetermined as much by the strain involved as by the cow factors already alluded to. This may also mean that the outcome of a treatment protocol is, to a significant extent, effectively determined by factors such as strain type and cow factors and not by the drug or protocol itself. This may go some way to explain why a successful outcome in *Staphylococcus aureus* treatment in the dry period, let alone during lactation, is so difficult to both predict and achieve.

Coagulase-negative Staphylococci

Coagulase-negative *Staphylococci* (CNS) species are frequently isolated from bovine milk samples. However, it is not always clear whether they have originated from the teat or udder skin or from within the gland itself. In general, they are viewed as skin commensals, but some species do have the potential to colonize the teat canal. They are often referred to as a minor pathogen (along with other potential commensal bacteria such as *Coynebacterium bovis*), which implies that they are either mildly pathogenic or non-pathogenic. CNS infections are present in between 10 and 20 per cent of quarters, with infections being more common in early lactation. However, this high prevalence in early lactation will generally decline in the first few weeks after calving

---

Key Points

- Considered to be a normal teat skin/udder commensal
- Cattle are main source of infection
- Mildly contagious – can spread from cow to cow
- Clinical cases do occur but are not common
- Sub-clinical infection is common, particularly in fresh calved heifers
- Infections often self-cure
- Control – five-point plan, good milking routine.

Laboratory Characteristics

- Grows on blood agar
- 3–4mm oil-drop colonies
- Colonies generally white on blood agar and generally non-haemolytic
- Gram-positive cocci, *see* photo on page 154
- Catalase-positive, *see* photo on page 154
- Coagulase-negative, *see* photo on page 155
- Some coagulase-negative strains can have haemolysis typical of *Staphylococcus aureus* and may be best assumed to be potentially *Staphylococcus aureus* despite being coagulase-negative.

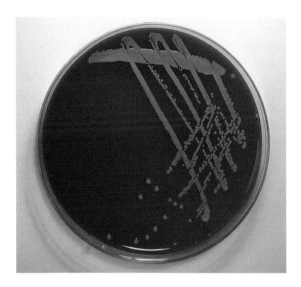

CNS cultured on blood agar.

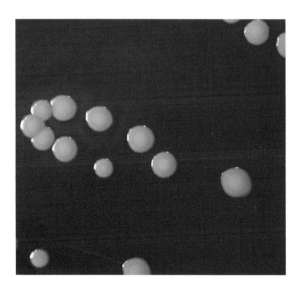

White oil-drop colonies typical of CNS.

as a result of self-cure. It is not clear why cows are commonly infected and then self-cure, but the flushing effect of milking may well play a part. As a result of these 'natural' fluctuations CNS cannot be classified as either contagious or environmental.

CNS may afford some protection to quarters against subsequent infection in a non-specific way by elevation of SCC or more specifically against *Staphylococcus aureus*. However, it appears that CNS do not provide protection against infections by environmental pathogens or *Streptococcus agalactiae*.

Laboratory differentiation between *Staphylococcus aureus* and coagulase-negative *Staphylococci* is by a positive reaction to the coagulase test. The specificity of the commonly used latex agglutination version of this test is approximately 97 per cent, and so some *Staphylococcus aureus* cultures can test as coagulase-negative. Consequently, it may be best to assume that *Staphylococci* that have the typical alpha beta haemolysis commonly associated with *Staphylococcus aureus* but test coagulase-negative may, in fact, be *Staphylococcus aureus*.

Culturing CNS from a milk sample will not always indicate that there has been an inflammatory reaction in the mammary gland, for example, an increased SCC, and may not even indicate intramammary infection. The possibility of transfer to the milk sample from teat or udder skin during the sampling procedure cannot always be ruled out. A good sampling protocol will help reduce the potential of contamination of milk samples with CNS from teat or udder skin when samples are being taken. A positive culture from repeated sequential sampling makes a stronger case for true intramammary infection and helps rule out other bacterial causes which may have been missed on a single sample, particularly if the SCC is elevated throughout the sampling sequence, adding to the belief that there is a significant persistent infection present. CNS are of low pathogenicity and consequently, although clinical cases can occur, sub-clinical infection is far more common. It is probably best to view the inflammatory responses to CNS as being the result of the bacteria getting the upper hand and being present in sufficient numbers to challenge the immune system, such that the SCC rises. Despite this, the rise in SCC at a quarter level, particularly if the infections are mild and sub-clinical, can often be relatively minor. Equally, when these mild quarter infections are considered at a cow level, where composite samples are measured, the increase in SCC may be close to insignificant. However, where the prevalence is high and where many cows have multiple quarter sub-clinical infections or cows have more significant infections, the effect on increasing BMSCC can be demonstrable. It is also worth remembering that, despite their low pathogenicity, CNS infections can occasionally contribute to clinical cases of mastitis in dairy herds, but are rarely a major cause.

Streptococcus agalactiae

Streptococcus agalactiae or Lancefield's Group B *Streptococcus* (GBS) was first reported as a cause of bovine mastitis in 1887 [Nocard and Mollereau, 1887]. *Streptococcus agalactiae* is an obligate udder pathogen, which means that it has difficulty surviving outside the udder and is perhaps therefore the most contagious of the contagious mastitis pathogens. Due to the fact that survival outside the udder in the dairy cows' environment is rare, its presence in a herd can be readily controlled by good parlour hygiene. However, the corollary of this is that a *Streptococcus agalactiae*-free herd can become infected by inadvertently purchasing an infected cow. Application of the five-point plan will, in many cases, facilitate eradication from the herd over time, although treatment of either the infected cows (partial blitz) or the whole

> ### Key Points
>
> - Can be eradicated from a herd
> - Identify infected herds by sampling bulk milk or cows with high SCCs
> - Cattle are almost exclusively the source of infection
> - Clinical cases are easy to treat
> - Sub-clinical cases more common
> - Generally increases SCC dramatically, but *Streptococcus agalactiae* is not restricted to herds with very high cell counts
> - Contagious – spreads easily from cow to cow
> - Risk factors – purchase of infected cattle
> - Control – five-point plan, good milking routine and vigilant use of antibiotic for all clinical cases and all cows at drying off.

herd (total blitz) can be used to accelerate the process. Many dairy herds in the developed world would expect to have a *Streptococcus agalactiae*-free status. However, there are still herds where this pathogen has not been eliminated and the effect on the cell count of infected cows is generally significant. In

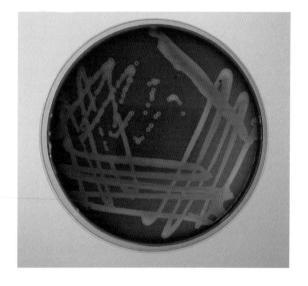

Streptococcus agalactiae cultured on blood agar, viewed on an X-ray viewer screen; note the clear beta haemolysis.

Laboratory Characteristics

- Grows on blood agar and Edwards agar
- 1–2 mm smooth, translucent, convex colonies
- Colonies blue white on Edwards agar – particularly under UV light
- NAS Strep (Non-Aesculin Splitting Streptococci)
- Other NAS Streps such as *Streptococcus* (now *Gemella*) *morbillorum*, *Streptococcus acidominimus*, *Streptococcus diacetyl lactis* and *Streptococcus lactis* can be mistaken for *Streptococcus agalactiae* by the unwary, although they are not Lancefield Group B and, in the author's experience, they are isolated infrequently and never as a herd problem
- Generally beta haemolytic – clear haemolysis, particularly visible on blood agar
- Gram-positive cocci; *see* photo on page 154
- Catalase-negative; *see* photo on page 154
- Lancefield Group B.

those herds where several cows are infected a recycling of infection will take place within the milking herd. The route of transmission is by the spread of contaminated material on milkers' hands or via the milking machine. *Streptococcus agalactiae* can cause clinical mastitis. However, infected herds do not often have excessive clinical mastitis rates and those cases which do occur are often mild and the response to antibiotic therapy is usually good. *Streptococcus agalactiae* more often presents as a hidden infection and an important cause of sub-clinical mastitis in infected herds, and, if left uncontrolled, will often result in the elevation of a significant number of individual cow cell counts, which, in turn, can elevate the bulk tank cell count, resulting in financial penalties for the herd.

The ease with which *Streptococcus agalactiae* clinical cases can be treated is paralleled by the virtually 100 per cent efficacy of antibiotic dry cow therapy in eliminating the infection from infected cows. However, in endemically infected herds the bacteria survive within the milking cow population by spreading readily between milking cows and, despite the fact

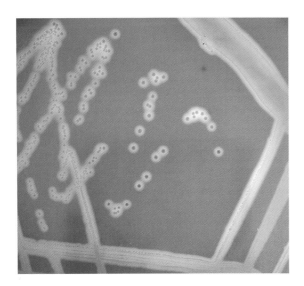

Streptococcus agalactiae, zoomed-in photo showing beta haemolysis.

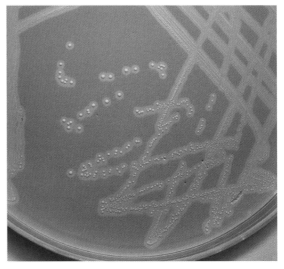

Streptococcus agalactiae cultured on Edwards media, viewed under ultra-violet light, again the clear beta haemolysis can be easily seen.

that individual cows are cleared of infection by antibiotic dry cow therapy, they soon become reinfected from these infected milking cows once they calve and rejoin the milking herd. Cows infected with *Streptococcus agalactiae* will often have only one infected quarter, but it is not uncommon for multiquartered infections to occur, especially in cows from herds where the infection has been endemic for a number of years. Infected cows will invariably have elevated cell counts at some stage of their sub-clinical infection. Some cows will become clinical and then cell counts can rise significantly. Generally, management is poor on these long-term infected herds and clinical mastitis detection is such that the difference between clinically and sub-clinically infected cows becomes blurred. Treatment is often delayed and consequently infection spreads more readily, and some cows have very high cell counts. Individual cell counts (ICCs) of 1,000,000 to 2,000,000 cells/ml are not unusual. However, both the ICC and the excretion of bacteria in the milk can vary considerably. ICCs >200,000 per ml are now generally accepted as an indicator of sub-clinical infection. The author has had experience of cows with positive *Streptococcus agalactiae* and an ICC of <150,000 cells/ml where samples were taken on the same day. Intermittent excretion is also a feature of *Streptococcus agalactiae* infection (as it is for staphylococcal infections). Two cows on one problem herd investigated by the author were sampled daily for six days and one cow actually became culture-negative on one day. This obviously has implications when performing herd screens to check for individual infected cows.

Infection is almost always introduced by purchased cattle. In *Streptococcus agalactiae*-infected herds where the BMSCC has been elevated for some years, the infection is often widespread and endemic. However, in herds which are closely monitored it is possible to pick up the infection soon after an introduction into the herd, either by being alerted by rising BMSCC or by isolating *Streptococcus agalactiae* from routine bulk milk bacteriological monitoring.

In the author's practice many herds' bulk milk is regularly bacteriologically screened every three months.

Approach to a Herd Where *Streptococcus agalactiae* Has Been Identified

The isolation of *Streptococcus agalactiae* is always significant and dairy herds should aim to maintain a *Streptococcus agalactiae*-free status. The infection may have been isolated from a routine monitoring bulk milk sample or, in the case of a high BMSCC herd investigation, from either a bulk milk or an individual high SCC cow (or quarter) sample.

There are broadly three approaches:

1. Total herd blitz – treat all quarters of all cows with antibiotic simultaneously, using milking cow or dry cow therapy as appropriate;
2. Partial herd blitz – identify and treat only infected cows;
3. Rely totally on good dairy management practices (for instance, NIRD five-point plan) to control and eventually eradicate the infection.

The choice of approach will depend, not only upon the current financial losses being suffered as a result of the *Streptococcus agalactiae* infection within the herd, but also the recent herd history in terms of BMSCC and recent cow purchases (if any). Any financial losses will clearly depend on the prevalence of *Streptococcus agalactiae* infection (how widespread?) within the herd, which, in turn, will be linked to both the clinical mastitis rate (direct costs) as well as the generally more significant losses from elevation of BMSCC (indirect costs). The indirect costs resulting from increased SCCs, at both the cow and the herd level, will be from both obvious losses from financial penalties from the first-time buyer (deducted from the 'milk cheque') as well as the less obvious in terms of reduced yield and quality. There is, of course, a big difference between a herd with a BMSCC of, say, <100,000 cells/ml and well within the top milk quality payment band where *Streptococcus agalactiae* has been isolated from a bulk sample, and a herd with a BMSCC in excess of the EU limit of 400,000 cells/ml and with, say, 30 per cent of the herd identified as *Streptococcus agalactiae*-infected. When one considers that it is likely that the herd with a BMSCC <100,000 cells/ml will have a good milking routine and, therefore, not only is the chance of spread within the herd much reduced, but, as there are no financial milk price penalties being incurred, there is no incentive to take action in any way other than to be extra diligent in the milking routine to ensure the likelihood of spread within the herd continues to be minimized. However, the herd with a BMSCC in excess of the EU 400,000 cells/ml limit is under some pressure not only to reduce the BMSCC to minimize, or ideally eliminate, any price penalties being incurred, but ultimately to ensure with some urgency that the milk is fit for human consumption or indeed is collected. It is in these situations that the cost benefits of blitz therapy start to make financial sense, mainly driven by the speed with which the BMSCC can be returned to

Pros and cons of total versus partial blitz therapy for the control of *Streptococcus agalactiae*

Total herd blitz	Partial herd blitz
High prevalence	Low prevalence
Chronically infected herd Long-term high BMSCC	Newly introduced/identified infection BMSCC only recently risen (or not even risen yet)
High proportion of herd in milk	Low proportion of herd in milk

NB If not using routine DCT ensure all cows currently dry receive milking cow antibiotic in **all four quarters** before they are milked (ideally just before they calve). Then start routine DCT programme.

More simple procedure May well be cheaper in the long run	Willingness and ability to follow protocol very carefully

Current financial situation
Calculate present payment losses per month (total litres sold × pence per litre penalty)
These losses can be considerable (£100s) even for small herds

Financial calculations ('Break even period')
Estimate herd cell count (BMSCC) response and calculate a *realistic* increase in monthly income from reduced payment penalties. Calculate the number of months of increased income required to recoup total treatment costs, **including value of discarded milk** during treatment

Milk withhold implications
Several cows are being treated with both partial and total blitz – it is advisable to notify the first-time buyer and get the bulk milk tested for inhibitory substances prior to collection

acceptable levels, often within a few days of treatment. Blitz treatment can be either partial (treatment of cows identified as infected with *Streptococcus agalactiae* only) or total (treatment of the whole herd). The decision of whether to use a partial herd or total herd blitz may well be influenced by the factors listed in the table on page 53.

Pros and Cons of Total versus Partial Blitz Therapy for the Control of *Streptococcus agalactiae*

The choice between partial or total blitz is very much a personal one and really hinges on the prevalence within the herd (i.e. how many cows are infected?). The apparent potential attraction of reduced costs (particularly fewer intramammary tubes required and less milk to discard) of a partial blitz may be more than wiped out by the need to repeatedly identify and treat infected cows in the herd. Bulk milk sampling twice a week while milk from known infected cows under treatment during a partial blitz is being withheld can give an indication if other infected cows exist in the herd. Intermittent excretion of bacteria and variable elevation of SCC may mean that the sensitivity of detection may be such that the elimination of *Streptococcus agalactiae* can be protracted. Even with the best milking routine it is possible that *Streptococcus agalactiae* can spread during the delay between sampling the cows to identify the infected animals and the actual treatment. The work required and the attention to detail by both veterinarian and farmer mean that this form of partial blitz treatment is not to be taken on lightly. Both methods involve a significant investment in time, with the need for careful planning and meticulous drug administration, as well as the costs of the antibiotic therapy itself. With whole herd treatment this is considerable and needs careful planning to ensure that all lactating and dry cows are treated. If one infected quarter exists after whole herd treatment, for example as a result of not receiving treatment, the infection may well spread within the herd and all efforts will have been in vain. A herd with a failed blitz

is no better than a herd which has undertaken no treatment. In fact, it is worse off as money has been 'wasted' on antibiotic treatment and milk has been discarded as a result. The practical task of treating all cattle with intramammary antibiotic in a hygienic manner should not be underestimated. There are always risks in terms of adverse effects, as well as benefits with any form of treatment and intramammary treatment is no different. The risks of some of these adverse effects tend to become more significant when whole herd treatment is undertaken. The infusion of antibiotic via the streak canal carries a number of risks, including damage to the normal defence mechanisms resulting from the physical trauma of introducing the end of the intramammary tube, the potential of inadvertently introducing contaminant bacteria or yeast, and the potential effects that broad spectrum antibiotics may have on the normal flora of the mammary gland, which may facilitate the development of infections by pathogens other than *Streptococcus agalactiae*, again such as yeast. There are reports of clinical cases of mastitis subsequent to treatment in herds where whole herd blitz has been undertaken and, in the light of this, the farmers need to be fully aware of the risks and appropriate emphasis placed on a good, clean infusion technique.

It must be realized that with a blitz approach the goal for the farmer and veterinarian will be different initially. As a result of the economic impacts of raised BMSCC on milk price the farmer will be looking for a reduction in BMSCC to achieve a better milk price as a return for the investment in time and drug. However the herds where *Streptococcus agalactiae* exists will often harbour other contagious mastitis pathogens, such as *Staphylococcus aureus* which cannot be eradicated from a herd with blitz antibiotic treatment. It is critical that samples are taken from a number of high SCC cows to establish the prevalence of other contagious pathogens, such as *Staphylococcus aureus*, so that the farmer is forewarned that the goal of *Streptococcus agalactiae* eradication can and will be achieved, but that further work may be necessary to reduce BMSCC to an acceptable level. The veterinarian will be aiming for an initial and achievable goal of eradicating *Streptococcus agalactiae* from the herd. Once it has been established that *Streptococcus agalactiae* has been successfully eradicated from the herd, it will be essential to improve contagious mastitis control by means of a much longer-term approach based around the five-point plan. The economics of treatment around the world will vary and will be affected by the financial penalties incurred for producing milk with elevated cell counts and the overall price paid for each litre of milk.

Although *Streptococcus agalactiae* (GBS) is well recognized as a cattle mastitis pathogen, a recent publication discussed the strain variations and differing lineages seen in isolates from mastitis cases in cattle and human cases of neonatal death from GBS. The author went on to postulate that, although the chance of interaction was low and the pasteurization of

Streptococcus agalactiae **risk factors and control measures**

Risk factors	Control measures
Purchasing infected cows	Keep a closed herd. Biosecurity – purchase from known *Streptococcus agalactiae*-free herds or test cattle prior to purchase or treat with post-treatment checks
Partial or non-existent dry cow therapy	Use antibiotic DCT on all cows
Partial or non-existent post-milking teat disinfection	Commence effective post-milking teat disinfection
Inadequately maintained and serviced milking parlour	Biannual milking machine tests Liners replaced every 2,500 milkings
Inadequate recording and attention to detail	Implement mastitis and milk recording system
Unhygienic parlour practices (udder cloths, dirty hands etc)	Vigorous application of the 5 Point Plan
Poor diagnosis resulting in insufficient therapy of clinical cases – 'missed' clinical cases (enabling spread to occur)	Sampling high SCC cows to identify *Streptococcus agalactiae*-infected cows and more diligent observation (foremilking, in line detectors etc) to help identify clinical cases
Lack of regular herd monitoring	Regular bacteriological monitoring of bulk milk (every 3 months) and or regular individual cow SCC testing (monthly) with selected high SCC cows bacteriologically sampled

milk should virtually eliminate the risk, in fact current knowledge indicates that the world dairy industry has the ability to eradicate the pathogen from all dairy herds, and there can be little sustainable argument against immediately setting about the eradication of this infection from the global dairy herd.

Streptococcus dysgalactiae

Streptococcus dysgalactiae is often labelled an environmental *Streptococcus*, and perhaps it is in the truest sense of the word in that it is widely distributed in the cow environment rather than being closely associated solely with faecal contamination. Cows often become infected between milkings when teat ends come into direct contact with faeces or soiled bedding, or at milking time, particularly when

poor udder preparation occurs prior to milking unit attachment. *Streptococcus dysgalactiae* is also often associated with poor teat condition and will be found commonly on sore or chapped teats or in herds suffering from blackspot. It is thought that in problem cases, where apparent response to treatment is poor, that this may be because of reinfection from the infected teat sore rather than any difficulty in treating the intramammary infection itself. *Streptococcus*

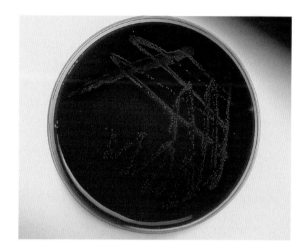

Streptococcus dysgalactiae cultured on blood agar viewed in natural light. Note the alpha (partial) haemolysis resulting in greening of the plate; the colonies have a target appearance.

Key Points

- Environmental with some contagious spread
- Associated with poor teat condition/sores
- Risk factors – poor milking time hygiene
- Clinical cases relatively easy to treat
- Sub-clinical infection does occur
- Control – five-point plan, good milking routine.

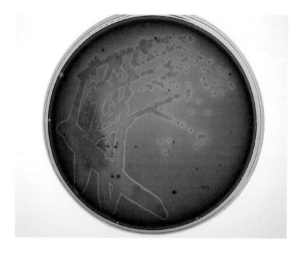

Streptococcus dysgalactiae cultured on blood agar, viewed on an X-ray viewer.

Streptococcus dysgalactiae cultured on Edwards media, viewed on an X-ray viewer.

Streptococcus dysgalactiae risk factors and control measures

Risk factors	Control measures
Machine damage to teats	Correct functioning and well maintained milking machine. Use of emollient, applied to dry, cracked teats after milking
Poor teat condition – caused by calves being left on cows	Use of good quality teat dip and good coverage
Physical teat damage, when teats are stood on	Pay attention to lame cows
Inadequate dry cow therapy	Correct and consistent use of DCT

Laboratory Characteristics

- Grows on blood agar and Edwards agar
- 1–2mm smooth, translucent, convex colonies
- Colonies are hard, non-viscid and can be pushed across the agar plate
- Generally alpha – (partial) haemolysis (greening) – with colonies often having a 'target' appearance
- Gram-positive cocci; *see* photo on page 154, Chapter 6
- Catalase-negative; *see* photo on page 154, Chapter 6
- Lancefield Group C

dysgalactiae, like most *Streptococci*, is more often than not sensitive to penicillin and antibiotic resistance is not generally a problem. Clinical cases caused by *Streptococcus dysgalactiae* tend to be sporadic and relatively easy to treat, but some infections do become persistent, which can result in an elevated SCC. Although contagious spread does occur, particularly with persistent infections, *Streptococcus dysgalactiae* is rarely sufficiently prevalent in a herd to elevate BMSCC. *Streptococcus dysgalactiae* can also be isolated from cases of summer mastitis as a component in the mixed bacteria complex, including *Arcanobacter pyogenes* (formerly *Corynebacterium pyogenes*), *Peptococus indolicus* and a miro-aerophilic micrococcus.

Streptococcus uberis

Streptococcus uberis has traditionally been regarded as an environmental pathogen; however, in some parts of the world the dairy industry has increasingly seen evidence that this pathogen can behave in a contagious manner. Evidence for this is based on not only field evidence but also strain-typing data, which tend to support the fact that, in parts of the world such as New Zealand, multiple strains are seen many of which, in all probability, originate from the dry period, supporting an environmental source. There will, of course, also be the possibility that

Key Points

- Sometimes called a faecal *Streptococcus*, particularly in the USA
- Originally seen mainly as an environmental pathogen
- More recently identified to have contagious risk
- Straw yards seen as a significant risk factor
- Causes both clinical cases and elevation of SCCs
- Persistent infections can occur
- Control – hygienic environment and five-point plan, good milking routine including pre- and post-milking dipping.

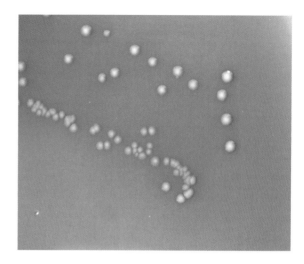

Streptococcus uberis cultured on Edwards media viewed on an X-ray viewer; note the aesculin splitting around the colonies.

Laboratory Characteristics

- Grows on blood agar, Edwards and selective media such as McConkey's
- 1–2mm smooth, translucent, convex colonies
- Generally non-haemolytic or alpha – partial haemolysis (greening)
- Aesculin-splitting, resulting in destruction of the purple colour of the Edwards media, which is more obvious when viewed as a lack of fluorescence under UV light
- Colonies often surrounded by a brown ring, unlike other aesculin-splitting faecal streptococci such as *Streptococcus bovis* or *Streptococcus faecalis* which is often surrounded by a black ring (now renamed *Enterococcus faecalis*)
- Gram-positive cocci (*see* photo on page 154)
- Catalase-negative (*see* photo on page 154)
- Heterogenous with respect to Lancefield typing and so cannot be assigned to any Lancefield group.

intramammary infection takes place in lactating cattle between milkings, as with any other environmental mastitis pathogen. However, in other parts of the world, such as the United Kingdom and the USA, there are often a few strains involved at a herd level with persistent infections occurring more commonly, which clearly will result in an increased chance of contagious spread.

This has considerable significance when determining treatment protocols for both clinical cases as well as the herd approach for treating high SCC cows. The chance of an infection spreading from cow to cow influences the cost-benefit calculations of treating sub-clinical (high SCC) mastitis. With strains of *Streptococcus uberis,* which have a net reproductive rate of >1, the chance of spread is higher and the benefit to the herd is greater, while those with a net reproductive rate <1 where contagious spread is unlikely little is to be gained by treating high SCC cows. The term 'cow-adapted' strains has been used to describe those strains that are more suited to growing in milk and setting up an infection.

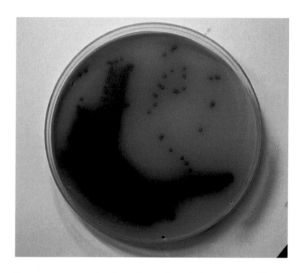

Streptococcus uberis cultured on Edwards media viewed under ultra-violet light; the aesculin splitting is more obvious.

The ability for a strain to break down proteins in milk, such as casein, to release free amino acids for their own nutrition gives a survival advantage such that they can multiply rapidly enough to establish as an infection rather than being flushed out by the effects of milking. Research work is on-going to look at strain variation, with a view to trying to identify not

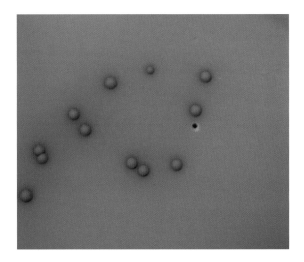

Streptococcus uberis, zoomed-in photo showing aesculin splitting around individual colonies.

only the variability in the ability for contagious behaviour, but also the genetic markers for this behaviour, if they exist. This research will potentially have two practical outcomes – identifying potential vaccine candidates and giving the ability to predict the likely behaviour characteristics of predominant strains found in a herd. The holy grail of a vaccine has to date been somewhat elusive, but the current concepts seem to be to try to interfere with the nutrition of the *Streptococcus uberis* bacteria. Clearly, as with any mastitis vaccine a cellular immune response, which would result in an increase in SCC, would be unacceptable to the dairy industry because of the deleterious effect on milk quality payment. There are a number of ways to convey a protective effect without producing an adverse SCC effect, including preventing the adherence and to some extent internalization of *Streptococcus uberis* to mammary epithelial cells by *Streptococcus uberis* adhesion molecule (SUAM) by directing antibodies at SUAM, improving the immune system response or effectively starving the *Streptococcus uberis* bacteria by targeting a unique part of its bacterial nutrition pathway.

Proof of this concept has been demonstrated by research targeting PauA, an enzyme used by *Streptococcus uberis* to break down casein into amino acids, facilitating *Streptococcus uberis* survival in milk, and stimulating cattle to produce antibodies to this essential protein. Although the concept is sound and some protection is afforded to experimental challenge, vaccinal response does not afford protection to all heterologous (different from the vaccinal strain) strains. Like the J5 *Escherichia coli* core vaccine, it seems that a *Streptococcus uberis* vaccine is likely to result in a reduction in severity rather than actually to prevent intramammary infection. Additionally for a vaccine to have a place in the commercial dairy industry it will need to afford a degree of protection across a broad range of *Streptococcus uberis* strains. Research is continuing to identify a suitable *Streptococcus uberis* vaccinal strain and a biochemical or genetic site for a vaccine target.

The study of strain types may also result in a useful practical tool for the veterinary surgeon in farm practice. If the ability of a *Streptococcus uberis* strain to survive and persist in a mammary gland is significantly related to the strain characteristics rather than to just the cow or environmental factors and this trait can be linked to an identifiable genetic marker within the bacteria, then a tool could be developed to effectively predict the likely potential for that strain to behave in a contagious manner. This information could be used for health planning by, say, checking the predominant strains of *Streptococcus uberis* found in a herd on a quarterly basis and using those data to indicate where the most common source of *Streptococcus uberis* was for that herd. This could be used to introduce or modify management practices which would impact on the chances of either environmental or contagious sources of *Streptococcus uberis* resulting in new intramammary infections. However, this does assume that the ability of any *Streptococcus uberis* strain to persist in the udder is strain-related and does not relate to cow factors, such as the ability of the cow to eliminate the infection. So has *Streptococcus uberis* changed or are cow factors more important? Have these persistent strains always been present or has *Streptococcus uberis* become cow-adapted? There are two schools of thought – either that these strains have developed in recent years or, more likely in the author's opinion, these carrier cows have always existed and persistent infections are not new but we now notice them with increasing frequency. The dairy industry has improved milk quality significantly over the last few decades and this is in no small part due to the improvements in hygienic milk production. These improvements have resulted in a significant reduction in faecal contamination of the udder resulting in not only improved bacterial counts in milk but also a significant reduction in the challenge to the teat end and reducing the chance of intramammary infections.

Historically, when the environmental challenge relating to *Streptococcus uberis* intramammary infection was perhaps more significant than it is now, any carrier cows with persistent infections were probably not only less obvious than they are now but also probably less significant overall in terms of herd infection. Over time, as the environmental source has been reduced, this has resulted in the increased significance of carrier cows with persistent infections such that these cows in some herds can now contribute a significant infection threat for the rest of the herd. Various 'fingerprinting' techniques can be used to differentiate a persistent infection where a consistent strain is isolated from an infected quarter over time, implying a persistent infection as compared to a repeat infection (cure followed by a reinfection), where different strains would be isolated at different time points. However, in the former situation it is also possible that a cure took place followed by a reinfection with the same strain, but one can be certain that in the latter situation that reinfection has occurred.

Strain-typing Methods

Most genetic fingerprinting techniques are based on either chopping the bacterial DNA into shorter lengths (restriction), the amplification of certain parts of bacterial DNA by means of polymerase chain reaction (PCR) or a sequential combination of both. The resulting DNA fragments have an electrical charge and will, depending on their size, move through a gel under the influence of an electrical field at varying speed. This allows the separation of the various fragments, resulting in a typical banding 'DNA fingerprint' pattern. These fingerprinting techniques are useful discriminatory tests to identify the same strain or to distinguish between different strains. Variations in these restriction (chopping of DNA) techniques have resulted in a number of recognized methods, including restriction enzyme analysis (REA), random amplified polymorphic DNA (RAPD), multi-locus sequence typing (MLST), random fragment length polymorphism (RFLP), pulsed-field gel electrophoresis (PFGE), and ribotyping.

MLST has recently been adopted as the world standard method for *Streptococcus uberis* strain typing, resulting in consistent genotype mapping and facilitating collaboration by research workers around the world which may speed up the development of the so far elusive effective *Streptococcus uberis* vaccine.

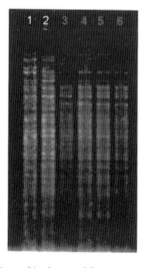

Strain typing of isolates of Streptococcus uberis showing persistent infection. Lanes 1 and 2 were from two different cows. Lanes 3–6 were serial samples from one cow with a a persistent infection that failed to respond to conventional treatment.

Strains can also be distinguished at a phenotypic level (that is, what they look like). Examples of this would possibly be by direct observation of colony characteristics as the colonies grow differently on the various agar plates, such that visual appearance of haemolysis or aesculin splitting on Edwards agar plates, or perhaps even antibiotic sensitivity patterns, may be used in differentiation.

Using these genetic strain typing techniques, persistent infections have been identified by a number of workers such that infections can be shown to persist throughout a lactation and even through a dry period and into the next lactation. However, despite this ability of some strains of *Streptococcus uberis* to become persistent infections, it is believed that in lactation 60 per cent of infections will last less than thirty days and only 18 per cent will become chronic and last in excess of a hundred days. It is worth remembering that in early lactation there is often more faecal contamination of cows and beds and so infection rates with environmental pathogens tend to be higher at this time.

What Are the Practical Upshots of Strain Typing if it Pans Out?

1. Persistent infections demonstrated by sequential sampling and strain typing.
2. Predictive strain typing has not been demonstrated to distinguish contagious and environmental strains, but this may be possible in the future.
3. If a genetic marker was identified to predict the ability to become persistent and therefore have an increased opportunity to behave in a contagious manner, then this differentiation could be used as part of a health planning process to modify management techniques, which would influence new infection rates with either contagious or environmental pathogens.

Although there is little doubt that several workers have shown sequential sampling indicating that certain strains have been shown to be persistent, and so have an increased chance of eliciting contagious behaviour for no other reason than that the longer duration of infection gives more opportunities to spread.

If a *Streptococcus uberis* that has been demonstrated to be contagious is put in another cow however, will it behave in a contagious manner?

The sources and characteristics of *Streptococcus uberis* are:

Environmental

- Source – straw, dung, soil and non-udder sources such as the skin and nose – straw yards are generally a greater risk than cubicles but a well managed straw yard can be better than less well managed cubicles
- Strain numbers – strain heterogeneity within herds, that is, many strains
- Animals infected – non-lactating animals such as heifers and dry cows, although cases may be later in the lactation
- Control – no eradication with five-point plan
- Antibiotic – dry cow therapy and internal teat sealants in dry cows with pre-milking teat disinfection within milking herd if environmental challenge continues after calving.

Contagious

- Source – other intramammary infections with risk increasing with persistent infections
- Strain numbers – more homologous (that is, fewer strains) with predominant strains within herds
- Animals infected – lactating animals more commonly infected
- Control – five-point plan; milking-time hygiene can significantly reduce new infection rates, including a significant effect of post-milking teat disinfectants (compare pre-milking disinfection).

Control measures for *Streptococcus uberis* within a herd will vary depending on whether environmental or contagious strains

Streptococcus uberis risk factors and control measures

Risk factors	Control measures
Warm, humid winter days favour survival of the organism. Poor ventilation and drainage of lactating and dry cow housing	Improve ventilation by creating inlets and outlets. Improve drainage by having sufficient slopes in cubicles (20cm fall front to back) and straw yards (1:60 towards feeding area)
Infrequent changes of straw bedding in yards (>5 weeks) and poaching around water troughs and gateways	Keep the bedding dry (quality storage, daily bedding, mucking out straw yards every three to five weeks where wet conditions are a problem) Move troughs to loafing areas
Over-stocked housing	Correct stocking density should allow 6.8m^2 for each 600kg cow
Fast-milking cows with large teat orifices	Genetic selection
Access to lying area within 30 minutes of milking	Let cows stand for 30 minutes after milking
Inadequate dry cow therapy. Failure to clear up existing infections at drying off will mean that the infection will persist through to calving	Use high quality appropriate DCT. Treat udder infections aggressively. Cull persistently infected cases
The overuse of calving paddocks – especially underneath trees	Move cattle
Contaminated teats	Pre-milking teat cleaning and disinfection Ensure hygienic parlour routine
Strep. uberis carrier cows – cows persistently infected with *Streptococcus uberis*	Early identification and repeated culture for bacteriology and sensitivity
Poor immunity	Include vitamin E/selenium in the ration

predominate. However, as with all mastitis, the NIRD five-point plan is important as a basis for control. More specific control measures which have found favour in a practical sense are pre-milking teat dipping and some form of protection for the rest of the herd from carrier cows combined with, where appropriate, the treatment of carrier cows to reduce the chance of spread. Pre-milking teat dipping has a number of effects, with perhaps the most repeatable being on milk hygiene. The effect of the disinfection of the teat surface prior to milking will be a reduction of the bacterial load on the teat skin which will, in turn, have beneficial effects on the hygiene of the milk produced. There is also a potential that, by reducing the number of bacteria on the teat skin prior to milking, the chance of these bacteria gaining entry to the quarter will be similarly reduced. This reduction in challenge to the teat end is likely to reduce the risk of mastitis at both a sub-clinical (elevated SCC) and a clinical level. Prevention of the spread of *Streptococcus uberis* to other uninfected cows in the milking parlour is no different from the approach with other contagious pathogens such as *Staphylococcus aureus*.

What Do We See Practically?

Clinical mastitis and sub-clinical mastitis (cows with increased SCC).

Many herds have what we might see as 'normal' mastitis cases which recover with antibiotic treatment. Some herds then appear to get problems with cases not responding to treatment with, perhaps, certain quarters being over represented. This may indicate that persistent infections are occurring. These can then drive infections in other cows in the same quarter, with the implication that it has spread contagiously. It is during this type of situation where treatment of high SCC infections can be beneficial.

Coliform bacteria

Coliform bacteria are sometimes grouped together as lactose-fermenting, Gram-negative, rod bacteria such as *Escherichia*, *Klebsiella*, *Enterobacter*, *Serratia* and *Citrobacter*, but may also perhaps incorrectly include non-lactose fermenting, Gram-negative, rod bacteria

---

Key Points

- Clinical cases vary from mild and self-curing to per-acute with toxic cases potentially resulting in the death of cow
- Can cause severe udder inflammation
- Sub-clinical infection is not common and unlikely to be associated with elevation of BMSCC
- Environmental – generally from faecal contamination of teat end
- Risk factors – poor hygiene and dirty housing and bedding
- Control – improve general hygiene, good milking routine.

Laboratory Characteristics

- Grow on blood agar and selective media such as McConkey's
- 2–5mm mucoid grey white colonies
- Can be either haemolytic or non-haemolytic
- Gram-negative rod
- Lactose fermentor resulting in pink colonies on McConkey agar
- Further distinguished by biochemical tests to *Escherichia coli*, *Klebsiella*, *Enterobacter*, *Serratia* and *Citrobacter*.

---

such as *Pseudomonas*, *Proteus* and *Pasteurella*. The most significant coliform mastitis-causing bacteria is *Escherichia coli* often shortened to *E. coli*.

Escherichia coli

E. coli is the most prevalent environmental mastitis-causing organism in the cow's environment and perhaps therefore not surprisingly the most common cause of environmental mastitis. It is present in faeces and soiled bedding in very large numbers, which increase dramatically when hygiene is poor. Wet, humid conditions both in housed cattle (where ventilation, stocking density, frequency and effectiveness of scraping out of passageways and general hygiene can influence infection rates) or when they are out at pasture (where inclement weather, either very wet or sometimes very hot, can influence infection rates) tend to increase the incidence of new intramammary infections. Poor ventilation and overcrowding in housing can increase the viability of *E. coli* allowing it to survive and multiply in the cow's environment resulting in a higher challenge at the teat end. The risks for *E. coli* mastitis are greatest just after drying off and just before calving, in common with other environmental pathogens. The risk around drying off is in some ways covered by dry cow therapy (depending on the product and the research work), while, until the advent of the internal teat seal such as Orbeseal, there was little

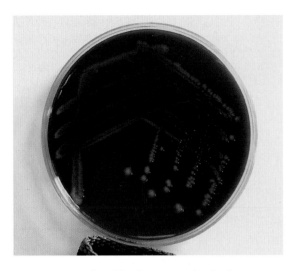

E. coli cultured on blood agar; notice the larger mucoid colonies.

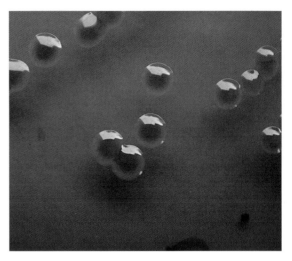

E. coli cultured on McConkey, zoomed-in photo showing pink mucoid colonies.

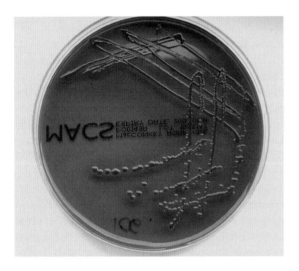

E. coli cultured on McConkey a selective media; the pink colonies indicate lactose fermentation by the colonies, which is typical of most Enterobacteriacae.

protection in the late dry period. Generally, *E. coli* infections are best seen as opportunistic invaders of the mammary gland and, as such, are generally short-lived. Often many of the changes seen in an infected quarter and, in fact, the cow if she becomes ill, are the result of a toxic effect resulting from the exposed polysaccharide cell wall, often called endotoxin, when the immune system destroys the invading bacteria. The importance of limiting this toxic effect is shown by the better responses to treatment observed when anti-endotoxic drugs such as non-steroidal anti-inflammatory drugs (NSAIDs) are used as part of the treatment protocol. In mild cases of *E. coli* mastitis the infection is generally self-limiting and, if a cow-side real-time diagnosis were possible, many of these cases would get better without antibiotic. However, as treatment has to be administered immediately and no such real-time test is available, all cases of clinical mastitis generally receive antibiotic.

Cows are continually having their mammary glands invaded by *E. coli* (and other bacteria) and eliminating them without any outward signs. Some may develop to a clinical mastitis while others may result in a short duration of inflammatory response to facilitate the elimination of the invading bacterium with only a transient SCC rise as evidence. Some intra-mammary infections with *E. coli* may result in a few clots or flakes seen at the next milking which have disappeared by the subsequent milking as self-cure has again dealt with the invader. However, sometimes the challenge is too much and a clinical case ensues often resulting in a hot, hard, swollen quarter with a watery, sometimes serous discharge (a clear

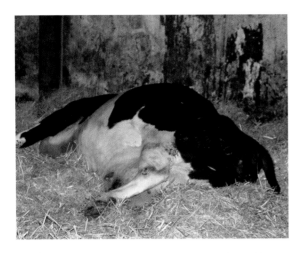

Recumbent cow suffering an acute toxic E. coli mastitis.

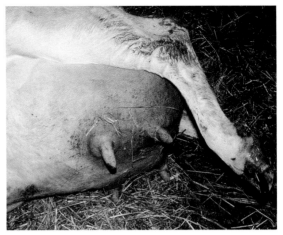

Udder from a cow suffering an acute toxic E. coli mastitis; note the discoloration of the udder from the toxic effect on the blood circulation.

yellow fluid like serum). Clinical *E. coli* mastitis typically occurs in early lactation, although the infection in many cases will have occurred in the dry period. *E. coli* mastitis can produce a variety of clinical signs, ranging from mild to very severe with some cases being fatal. Infections can occur in more than one quarter, but are not uncommon in more than one quarter, as befits an environmental pathogen, with the hindquarters being more commonly affected. Response to treatment depends on the severity of symptoms, the resistance of the cow and the promptness of therapy. The successful cow response is in part due to the cow's ability to produce white blood cells to fight the infection and some work in the late 1970s showed that if a cow could increase its SCC in the infected quarter within 4hr it was likely to survive, while those that were slow to respond allowed unchecked bacterial invasion and multiplication and were more likely to have severe symptoms or even die. This requirement for the multiplication of bacteria to overcome the immune system is common with environmental infections because, in general, they do not have the ability to adhere (stick) to the inner cells of the udder to avoid being flushed out by milk removal. For this reason chronic persistent infections resulting in repeated bouts

of mastitis are rare with environmental infections. However, recent work on fingerprinting has shown that persistent infections do occur: many infections in early lactation originate from a dry-period, new intramammary infection and on occasions persistent infections with *E. coli* can result in repeat cases and the elevation of SCC, although it is unlikely that this will be prevalent enough to affect BMSCC significantly.

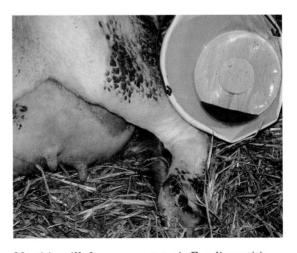

Mastitic milk from an acute toxic E. coli mastitis, showing bloody serum discoloration and consistency.

Escherichia coli risk factors and control measures

Risk factors	Control measures
Wet conditions. Contaminated or dirty bedding or environment (lying areas, collecting yards and gateways)	Keep the general environment clean and dry
Inadequate, dirty or wet bedding in calving and pre-calving housing (infection may enter udder in dry period and produce symptoms in early lactation/at calving)	Keep the general environment clean and dry, scrape cubicle passages at least three times daily
Insufficient number of calving boxes	Ensure sufficient number of calving boxes, and clean dry storage of bedding
Cramped or poorly designed straw yards (poached areas around troughs, entry points, inadequate ventilation etc.)	Improve ventilation/drainage and mucking out to reduce multiplication of bacteria (long term). Investigate stocking rate. Bed up frequently with clean dry 'barn stored' straw
Oestrus behaviour in housed cattle resulting in disturbed and dirty bedding. Cows bulling on slippery concrete will mean dirty udders	Remove bulling cows from straw yards
Poor cubicle design (too long or wide for heifers, too short for cows, resulting in lying out. Inadequate fall, raised lip on heel stone, inadequately placed brisket board or head rail causing dunging on the cubicle etc.)	Separate the udder from faeces by improving housing design and bedding (lying space, cubicle fit and design). Cubicle area should be at least 2.3m × 1.15–1.2m
Faulty milking machine function or design (small claw pieces, vacuum fluctuations within the claw, claw piece flooding)	Ensure that the parlour is functioning correctly Check machine annually and rectify faults
Washing teats and poor parlour hygiene (emulsifying faeces on teats prior to milking)	Check and improve parlour routines. Establish pre-milking teat disinfection
Open teat orifice (fast-milking cows, cows lying down too soon after milking)	Increase milking frequency (milk high-yielding cows every eight or twelve hours). Attention to cubicle design Ensure that milking cows stand for 30 minutes after milking
Damaged teats (teat trodden on, teat orifice damage)	Pay attention to lame cows – lame cows are more likely to lie down and get up awkwardly, increasing the risk of standing on their teats.

Escherichia coli **risk factors and control measures – cont.**

Risk factors	Control measures
Inadequate milking out of the udder (and running milk)	Check ACR function and parlour routine
Excessive udder development pre-calving and running milk	Pre-calving hygiene including teat dipping and attention to nutrition
Poor hygiene when infusing intramammary products	Ensure hygienic infusion technique

The control of *E. coli* is generally based around hygiene, optimization of the cow's immune response via good nutrition, and the possible use of vaccination; however, if persistent infections are found to be a problem in some herds and *E. coli* is becoming more adapted to the udder environment, then this may not be the total solution.

There is an *E. coli* J5 core oil adjuvant killed vaccine available in the United Kingdom (and the USA) to reduce intramammary infection caused by *E. coli*. The vaccine is given in three doses: at drying off, four weeks later and within two weeks after calving and will reduce the severity rather than totally prevent cases. Some veterinarians have found it to be a useful tool in the fight against *E. coli* mastitis. Particular attention to the dry cow and the time around (just before and just after) calving is essential to avoid a high clinical incidence in the early part of a cow's lactation. However, it is still fair to say that in a herd outbreak of clinical mastitis with *E. coli* many strains may be involved as there is a ready source of bacteria from the faecal contamination which is ubiquitous in the cow's environment.

Apart from strains of *E. coli* that cause clinical mastitis, there are non-pathogenic strains associated with cattle which can be found in milk that is not produced in a hygienic manner. Although of no clinical significance in cattle, there is the potential for the faecal contamination of milk by *E. coli* 0157:H7 which can be a significant human enteric pathogen. The hygiene of milk production relates closely to the potential contamination of milk.

Klebsiella
Klebsiella is an environmental organism commonly associated with damp and dirty housing and, in particular, with the contamination of wood-based products such as sawdust bedding. Research has shown that dairy cows commonly excrete *Klebsiella* with up to 80 per cent of faecal samples being positive in one study. In some outbreaks there has been some evidence of contagious spread.

Pseudomonas
Pseudomonas is a non-lactose fermenting, Gram-negative bacterium which can cause severe and sometimes chronic mastitis. The organism is strongly associated with water and, on occasions, has been associated with the contamination of water sources such as heated supplies for teat washing, especially if bore hole water is used without treatment or a sanitizing solution.

Proteus

Proteus deserves a special mention more for its ability as a contaminant rather than as a cause of mastitis. It is a non-lactose fermenting, Gram-negative bacterium found widely in the cow environment including bedding, feed and water. It can on occasion cause mastitis, but is perhaps more often associated with sample contamination, mainly because it is highly motile on blood agar and 'swarms' over the whole plate obscuring any other bacterial isolates and rendering the samples useless. It also produces a very characteristic and foul smell. However, it does not swarm on McConkey agar, where, as it is a non-lactose fermenter, it could be mistaken for *Salmonella* species which are themselves a rare cause of mastitis. The use of a urea slope will distinguish *Proteus* from *Salmonella*. In the author's experience, the isolation of *Proteus* is most often indicative of sample contamination. However, repeated culture from sequential samples would tend to indicate a true intramammary infection.

There are many other Gram-negative bacteria not listed above which can cause mastitis, including the lactose fermentors *Enterobacter*, *Serratia* and *Citrobacter* and the non-lactose

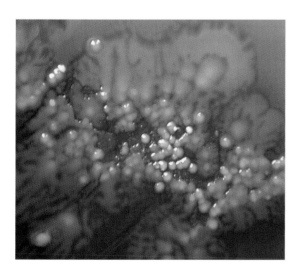

Proteus swarming on blood agar obscuring CNS colonies.

fermentor *Pasteurella* which are not uncommonly isolated from milk samples but are perhaps less likely to be involved in a herd problem.

Corynebacteria

These are a group of bacteria which are aerobic or facultatively anaerobic, irregularly shaped, non-spore forming, Gram-positive rods. The most commonly associated with the bovine mammary gland is *Corynebacterium bovis* which is lipophilic. There are a number of non-lipophilic members of this group which can on occasions cause mastitis in cattle. *Corynebacterium ulcerans*, which is perhaps the most notable of the non-lipophilic corynebacteria, also has an association with both non-bovine sources such as pets (in particular cats and dogs) and humans (patients with sore throats).

Corynebacterium bovis

Corynebacterium bovis is probably one of the most commonly isolated organisms cultured from bovine milk, although it is thought that it probably originates from the streak canal. It is highly contagious and spreads readily from cow to cow. Some work has shown a link to increased infection susceptibility with major pathogens while most work tends to show a reduced susceptibility. The 'protective' effect is thought to be via a number of possible routes, including competitive inhibition or even an antagonistic effect, perhaps via the production of an antimicrobial substance (bacteriocin). It is also possible that the stimulation of white cell production (increased SCC) in the quarter may induce some degree of increased resistance to infection. However, this may be only part of the protective effect as it seems to be more significant with *Corynebacterium bovis* than that seen with similar SCC elevation and coagulase-negative *Staphylococci*. In the 1970s work was done which used the herd prevalence of *Corynebacterium bovis* at various stages of the lactation as an indirect measure of the use of management practices such as post-milking teat disinfection and dry cow therapy. If

Corynebacterium bovis was highly prevalent in early lactation it was assumed that antibiotic dry cow therapy was not being used, and this situation can also sometimes be seen in organic herds.

If *Corynebacterium bovis* was highly prevalent in later lactation the implication was that post-milking teat disinfection was not being used effectively and cow-to-cow spread was readily occurring. Although *Corynebacterium bovis* can cause clinical mastitis on occasions, it is more an indirect measure of the potential for contagious spread within a herd. High prevalence of *Corynebacterium bovis* assumes more significance if other, more significant, major contagious pathogens such as *Streptococcus agalactiae*, *Staphylococcus aureus* or perhaps cow-adapted *Streptococcus uberis* are present in the herd. As a minor pathogen, the elevation of individual cow SCC can be minimal; however, if it is allowed to become sufficiently prevalent on a herd basis it can contribute to elevation of BMSCC.

Corynebacterium bovis is highly lipophilic, which means that it grows well in the fat found in milk and, as a consequence, is to be found in the primary streak on the agar plate where the milk fat tends to be concentrated, the colonies are small and often powdery and usually take 48hr to grow. This will mean that, when significant numbers of other pathogens are cultured on the plate, this bacterium can easily be missed as it is not very robust and can be 'choked' out. As a consequence, it is more often found in milk samples where few other bacteria are cultured.

Arcanobacter pyogenes

Arcanobacter pyogenes (formerly *Corynebacterium pyogenes* and *Actinomyces pyogenes* in between) can cause mastitis in its own right, but can also be isolated from cases of summer mastitis (*see* Chapter 9) as a component in the mixed bacteria complex along with *Streptococcus dysgalactiae*, *Peptococcus indolicus* and a miro-aerophilic micrococcus. *Arcanobacter pyogenes* is slow growing and the small colonies often take 48hr to become visible, but are generally surrounded by a very marked clear zone of haemolysis. In the author's experience mastitis caused by *Arcanobacter pyogenes* in pure culture can be difficult to treat despite being almost always penicillin-sensitive and systemic treatment in conjunction with intramammary tubes can help to improve cure rates. The

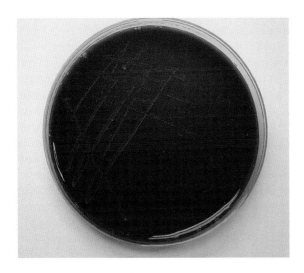

Corynebacterium bovis cultured on blood agar showing small, slow-growing powdery colonies.

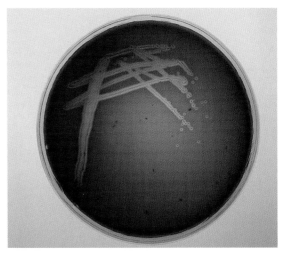

Arcanobacter pyogenes cultured on blood agar, showing typical clear haemolysis.

use of penethamate (Mamyzin; Boehringer Ingelheim) has appeared to improve cure rates in cases where intramammary tubes alone appear to have failed.

Bacillus spp.

Bacillus is a genus of rod-shaped, Gram-positive bacteria which are generally either obligate or facultative aerobes and include both free-living and pathogenic species. They are widespread in the environment and are found in soil, water, dust, air, faeces, vegetation, wounds and abscesses. Some *Bacillus* species under stressful environmental conditions can produce oval endospores that can stay dormant for extended periods. The best example of this type of spore formation would perhaps be *Bacillus anthracis* (anthrax). The culturing of *Bacillus* species, seen as large (up to 20mm) crusty colonies, are effectively a general description for soil contaminants which have been introduced into the milk during sampling. However, the introduction of Gram-positive bacilli into the udder often results from contaminated intramammary tubes or improper teat hygiene prior to intramammary treatment.

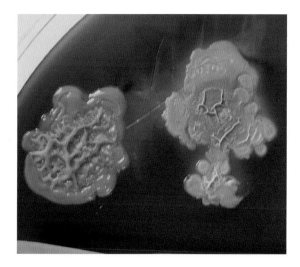

Bacillus species are often contaminant bacteria originating from soil or dirt.

Bacillus cereus

A proportion of clinical mastitis cases caused by *Bacillus cereus* may cause acute and sometimes fatal gangrenous mastitis. There appears to be an association in herds with multiple cases with the feeding of brewers' grains. *Bacillus cereus* is also responsible for a minority of human food poisoning instances (<5 per cent) and has been linked to the improper storage of cooked rice, but could be a zoonotic risk if raw milk is consumed. *Bacillus cereus* colonies are large, slightly grey with irregular edges and often surrounded by a clear zone of haemolysis.

Bacillus subtilis

Risk factors for *Bacillus subtilis* are similar to those for *Bacillus* species in general with respect to soil and feed as sources. *Bacillus subtilis* colonies are greenish-grey with a ground-glass appearance. Positive cultures, particularly in samples from high SCC cows, can be indicative of contamination during sampling rather than pointing to a causal pathogen.

Yeast

Yeasts such as *Candida* spp. are ubiquitous in the cow's environment and are most often opportunistic invaders of the udder. Yeast colonies are small, white and slow to grow generally, taking 48hr to appear, but can be cultured on blood agar. Under the microscope they are generally seen as large, ovaloid and Gram-positive and are often seen budding (replicating). Most herds will have sporadic and infrequent mastitis cases caused by yeast infections; however, there are some predisposing factors that can result in some herds having a particularly high incidence. The need for extended intramammary treatment protocols with difficult to treat mastitis cases found in some herds can increase the risk of yeast infection significantly. The repeated insertion of intramammary tubes through the streak canal will cause damage to the natural defence proteins and keratin which normally help to reduce the chance of pathogens invading the quarter. This, coupled with the risk

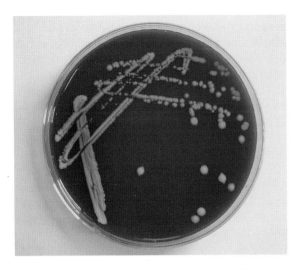

Yeast cultured on blood agar showing small, irregular, slow-growing colonies.

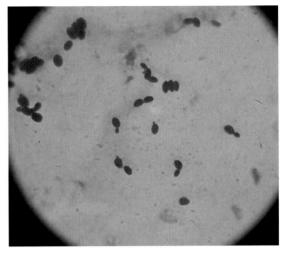

Yeast can be clearly seen under the microscope as budding fruiting bodies.

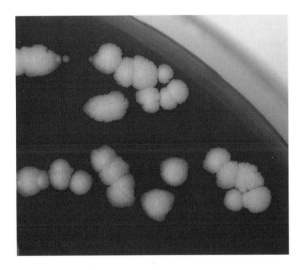

Yeast, zoomed-in to show irregular, rough colonies.

of physically introducing pathogens with the insertion of each tube, makes repeated tubing a significant risk for a yeast infection. When a case appears to fail to respond to prolonged antibiotic therapy, a yeast infection should be suspected. Because antibiotic has no effect on yeast infections, a milk sample for culture to check for a yeast infection can be taken even when antibiotic treatment is on-going. There are good reasons why a yeast infection needs to be identified as treatment will at best be

ineffective, but at worst continue to give the yeast a 'helping hand'. The negative effect of continued antibiotic therapy on the normal bacterial flora of the udder will remove competitive inhibition, often allowing the yeast to thrive. This can be further exacerbated in some cases as the stearate base found in many intramammary tubes can be nutritious for some yeast infections.

There are no licensed treatments for intramammary yeast infections; however, the use of a sterile solution of 1 per cent povidine iodine diluted to 3:1 (the author would use 50ml of iodine made up to 200ml with sterile water) infused at a rate of 20ml twice daily for five days can be effective. The use of a conventional 20ml syringe, provided that the nozzle is not inserted into the streak canal, can be quite adequate. The pressure of the thinner aqueous solution makes a non-insertion technique much easier than with, say, an antibiotic intramammary tube. The milk should be subjected to a milk inhibitory substance test such as Delvo SP (Gist Brocades) after a minimum statutory 'off-label', seven-day milk withhold period prior to the milk being returned to the bulk tank for human consumption. If identified early, the prognosis for a yeast mastitis is reasonable and the chance of treatment being successful certainly justifies the milk discard. A post-treatment check sample (seven to ten days after the last treatment) is advisable to ensure that the yeast has been successfully eliminated. There will be, however, a poor prognosis if the yeast infection is allowed to become established as chronic infections (as with any long-term intramammary infection) tend to cause udder damage and are more difficult to resolve.

Protatheca

An achlorophyllic alga which can also be an opportunistic pathogen, causing infections of the udder. More usually seen as an unresponsive clinical case, it can also result in sub-clinical mastitis with persistent elevation of SCC. As with yeast infections, antibiotic treatment will be completely ineffective and may, in fact, make things worse by removing bacteria representing the natural udder flora which could exert a competitive inhibition effect. Again, there is no treatment available, but the author has found iodine treatment, as described above in yeast infections, to be successful in some cases. The same milk withhold precautions apply.

Mycoplasma

Mycoplasma mastitis is not commonly diagnosed in the UK and is thought to be a rare cause of mastitis in the UK. This may in part be due to the fact that it is not always looked for in mastitis samples. *Mycoplasma* are sensitive to pH changes in milk, requiring a very fresh milk sample being delivered to the laboratory and special culture techniques. *Mycoplasma bovis*, *Mycoplasma californicum* and *Mycoplasma canadense* have all been associated with mastitis in the UK. *Mycoplasma bovis* is probably the most common and pathogenic form in the UK and is also associated with arthritis and lameness in cattle. As *Mycoplasma bovis* can be isolated from many non-udder sites, isolation from milk samples is not conclusive proof of true intramammary infection and can on occasions be an incidental finding, especially in herds suffering *Mycoplasma* lameness. Typically *Mycoplasma* mastitis fails to

respond to treatment and yeast or prototheca might also be suspected. Improved success has been observed with intramammary treatment with oxytetracyline (no longer available in the UK) or systemic treatment with either oxytetracycline or Tylosin (Tylan; Elanco Animal Health).

MASTITIS CONTROL PLANS

The approach to mastitis control may well vary around the world, but should, in general terms at least, encompass a holistic approach which addresses the host, environment and infectious agents. Despite the plethora of control plans that have been developed, they all have essentially only two basic elements; first, preventing new infections and, secondly, shortening the duration of any existing infections. So for example, preventing (or perhaps more realistically reducing) new infections would include both vaccination and a hygienic milking routine, while shortening the duration of existing infections would include both treatment and culling.

The approach to disease control will (and should) constantly evolve in response to knowledge from both practical experience and research. This will apply not only at the individual farm level but also within regions, countries and around the world. The first coordinated, worldwide mastitis plan was probably the 'five-point plan' in the 1960s from the National Institute for Research into Dairying (NIRD), *see* below. This plan came from a systematic and methodical appraisal of the then current knowledge of mastitis aetiology (causes) and epidemiology (spread). Once the major pathways and critical control points had been identified, the management practices most likely to have a significant controlling influence were identified and this was distilled down to a five-point plan. While the dairy industry has changed considerably since the time of the initial development of the five-point plan, the underlying structure of the plan still forms the basis of most modern mastitis control plans. Significant changes in the dairy industry resulting in a need for the modification of the original five-point plan would include changes to the types of cow, herd size and level of production, coupled with changes to the cow's surroundings.

The dairy industry, like much of food production after the Second World War, responded to a need for higher levels of production and greater efficiency. This drive within the industry resulted in a general increase in herd size coupled with a change in the type of dairy cow used for milk production. As a result, both the feeding and housing of dairy cows also changed. The traditional restrained housing (shippens or tie stall barns), where cows were housed and milked in the same accommodation, were replaced with free housing, including the introduction of systems such as cubicles and straw yards where the cows were milked in a milking parlour separate from the cow accommodation. These changes influenced the type and number of mastitis cases seen in dairy herds. As a consequence, the construction of mastitis control plans has evolved over the years, initially based on the then current knowledge base but being modified by developing knowledge. The development of a coordinated mastitis control plan was a great step forward by providing a uniform, logical approach within the industry using standard operating procedures (SOPs) targeted at areas where intervention was known to have a beneficial effect.

NIRD Five-point Plan

The five-point plan was devised in the 1960s and was aimed at giving the dairy industry a comprehensive action plan to control mastitis. The plan was aimed at both reducing new infections and reducing the duration of existing infections. The impact on new infections was by addressing the sources of infection, which, at that time, were mainly other cattle with infected quarters, together with fomite spread via the milking machine. Environmental infections, although less common at that time, have clearly assumed greater significance in recent years. Although the five-point plan is potentially weak in the control of infections of environmental origin, it is possible to upgrade the point regarding post-milking teat disinfection to 'hygienic teat management'. This then encompasses all the management factors required to present the cow in the milking parlour in the right condition to produce the high quality milk required by today's market. Many of the factors influencing new infection rates from environmental mastitis will, of course, relate to the cow's own environment. However, some will be direct and obvious like the hygiene and cleanliness of the housing and lying areas, while others will be just as significant but perhaps less obvious, such as ensuring that the diet is well balanced. The mechanism whereby the cow ration influences the mastitis new infection rate will be by ensuring that the rumen is functioning well and that there is sufficient fibre in the diet to achieve good faecal consistency. Cows fed a diet resulting in soft or diarrhoeic faeces will contaminate their environment, including their lying areas, their udders and teats, more readily, resulting in higher infection rates with bacteria such as *E. coli* or *Streptococcus uberis*.

Original Five-point Plan

1. Post-milking teat disinfection
2. Dry off all cows with antibiotic dry cow tubes
3. Treat all clinical cases promptly with antibiotic
4. Cull cows with persistent and repeat cases
5. Milking machine is to be serviced and maintained.

Modified and Updated Five-point Plan

1. **Hygienic teat management** Clean, dry, well-ventilated housing management combined with adequate teat preparation (with possible use of pre-milking teat disinfection) and post-milking teat disinfection. Present cow at parlour with udder and teats in appropriate condition to produce high quality milk required by today's market place.

2. **Abrupt drying off** (Not milked once a day.) Teat ends swabbed with spirit or medicated wipes and then tubed in a specific order. Clean furthermost teats first and the nearest teats next. Infuse tubes with dry cow preparation in the opposite order. (This avoids contaminating teat ends just prior to tubing.) Use most appropriate dry cow tube for the situation in terms of most prevalent bacteria, dry-period length and need to use either internal teat seal (Orbeseal; Pfizer Animal Health) or external teat seal (Dryflex; Deosan).
3. **Early detection** plus appropriate therapy and recording of all clinical mastitis cases. Computer recording systems make for easy analysis (such as Interherd). Use most appropriate milking cow tube in terms of most prevalent bacteria, plus, if necessary, adjunctive treatment to achieve bacteriological cure.
4. **Cull persistent offenders** Three cases in one quarter or five cases in mixed quarters in one lactation is a good rule of thumb in order to place the cow on the cull list.
5. **Use a milking machine capable of meeting modern hygienic milking requirements** This should be maintained in good working order. Service the plant twice or more yearly, depending on herd size and number of units. Liners should be changed approximately every 2,500 milkings.

National Mastitis Action Plan

There are other approaches towards updating the original plan. The National Mastitis Action Plan (Mastitis MAP) was developed by ADAS and VLA as part of a MAFF Animal Welfare Campaign and builds on the strength of the NIRD/CVL Five Point Mastitis Control Plan to more effectively control environmental infections. The Mastitis MAP (Defra Publication, PB4661) was launched in 1999.

The key elements of the Mastitis MAP are:

* Hygienic teat management
* Prompt identification and treatment of clinical mastitis
* Dry cow management and therapy
* Accurate record keeping
* Culling of chronically infected cows
* Regular milking machine maintenance and testing.

The National Mastitis Council (NMC) in the USA has created a ten-point mastitis control plan, where the extra points address the environmental factors and the need for recording, monitoring and target setting. There are various approaches to reducing the spread of infection from infected to uninfected cows within the parlour. The original five-point plan approach has direct and indirect impacts on infection spread within the parlour via all five points.

CHAPTER FOUR

The Milking Machine and Milking Routine

THE MILKING MACHINE

The milking machine harvests milk, the major source of income for a dairy farm, making it possible to keep and milk many more cows than if the milk were extracted by hand. Milking machines are generally used at least twice daily and for several hours at a time and so are probably one of the, if not the, most used pieces of equipment on a dairy farm. Despite this familiarity that dairy farmers have with their milking machines and the fact that they are generating their major income, they can at times be neglected in terms of day-to-day maintenance and regular servicing. The milking machine can have an effect on both mastitis and milk quality. The milking machine influence on mastitis can be both on existing infections by the exacerbation of them or by the facilitation of a new intramammary infection, resulting in either the elevation of SCC or the triggering of a clinical case. The milking machine influence on milk quality is mainly through the degree of bacterial contamination where a hygienic milking routine will influence mainly bactoscan.

History and Development

In its simplest form the removal of milk for human consumption from cows was by hand milking, although this is by positive pressure and is different from a calf sucking or milking machines which use negative pressure or a partial vacuum. The partial vacuum interferes with the blood flow to the teat, which soon becomes painful, much as when an elastic band is applied to a finger, and a constant vacuum, although tried in early milking machines, was soon replaced with a pulsating system of alternate vacuum and atmospheric pressure. Initial attempts to move away from hand milking in the 1800s comprised four simple metal tubes (cannulae) connected to a pail (bucket) which was suspended on a band around the cow's loins. Each cannula was inserted into a teat orifice and the milk flowed out under a combination of gravity and intramammary pressure. The first patent was granted to Blurton in 1836 and non-vacuum milking devices were sold up to around the time of the First World War. The fact that common cannulae were used between cows, spreading infection, coupled with the physical trauma to the important streak canal, meant that mastitis was common when using these devices.

Development of a vaccum-based system resulted in the first patent application from two British inventors Hodges and Brockedon in 1851. However, even with the advent of vacuum-based milking devices, the use of a band to support the receiver vessel persisted well into the twentieth century. The next significant advance was the development of a 'pulsator' in 1895 with the Thistle Milking Machine, where alternate vacuum and atmospheric pressure relieved the teats from constant vacuum, reducing congestion and allowing blood flow to be maintained to the teats. To this day these basic principles of milking-machine function remain unchanged and, while virtually all dairy cattle are now machine-milked (apart from open farms as tourist attractions), the proportions in the 1940s were as little as 10 per cent in the USA, 30 per cent in the United Kingdom and 50 per cent in Australia and New Zealand. Continued developments in terms of refinements, electronic control and automation of various elements of the milking routine have been considerable and are on-going. Much as the car is still running on an internal combustion engine, albeit with electronic fuel injection, which can be likened to the electronic pulsation control rather than the mechanical equivalents, the fundamental parlour design, like that of the car, is not dissimilar to that of a century ago.

BASIC DESIGN AND COMPONENTS

Entire books have been written on the milking machine and it is outside the scope of this one to become a milking-machine reference text. Nevertheless, a working knowledge of the machine is essential to understand its influence on mastitis and milk quality. There are many configurations for milking parlours, such as abreast, herringbone, trigon, auto-tandem and rotary, all having their own attributes and variations, such as the orientation or angle the cows stand at, as well as exit the parlour, such as rapid exit parlours. However, they all have the same basic components to allow milk to be harvested and the plant to be cleaned once all the cows have been milked.

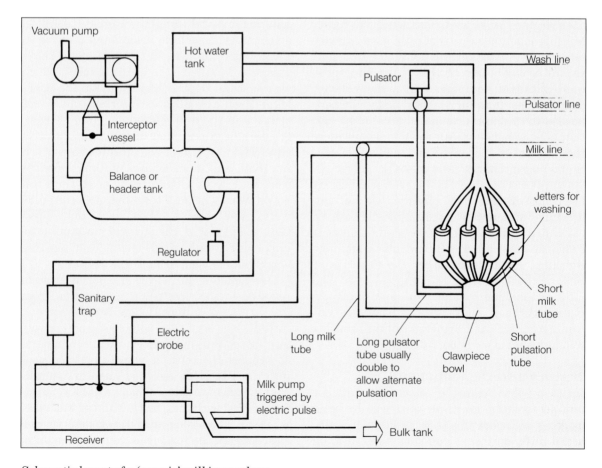

Schematic layout of a 'generic' milking parlour.

Vacuum Pump

An air pump which produces a partial vacuum in the entire milking system by extracting air and exhausting it to the atmosphere. The pump needs to have the ability to create a vacuum reserve by being able to extract more air than is necessary to run the milking machine, including any ancillary equipment such as gates, feeders and ACRs. As well as coping with air admissions, such as when units are attached to cows or if a unit were to fall off, the pump must be able to still maintain the vacuum at the desired level.

Interceptor Vessel

An interceptor vessel is situated in the main vacuum line between the vacuum pump and the sanitary trap to prevent liquid or foreign matter from reaching and damaging the pump.

Balance Tank or Header Tank

A vessel situated at the end of the main vacuum line (between the interceptor and the sanitary trap) with the milking and pulsation lines emanating from it and serving as a storage tank for vacuum and so effectively balancing or increasing the plant's reserve.

Sanitary Trap

A vessel with a floating ball valve situated between the milking and air systems to prevent contamination of liquid to the air system. Generally constructed of glass or plastic so it is transparent for easy visibility.

Regulator

An automatic valve designed to maintain a steady vacuum by admitting air to the main vacuum line. The amount admitted will depend on the current vacuum reserve, which will depend on other air admissions such as unit attachment, ACRs or the use of vacuum by gates and feeders. The regulator should be heard 'hissing' at all times, otherwise all the vacuum reserve has been used up.

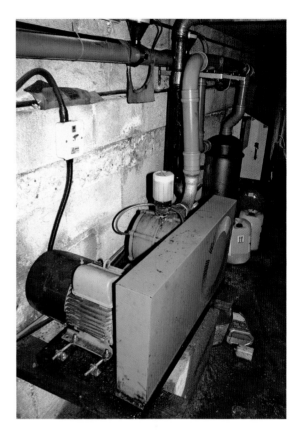

Vacuum pump.

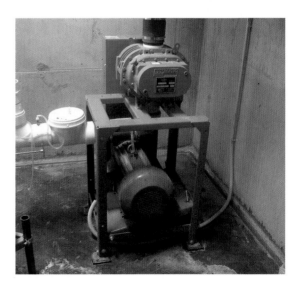

Variable speed vacuum pump, which 'works to demand' and is aimed at cost saving.

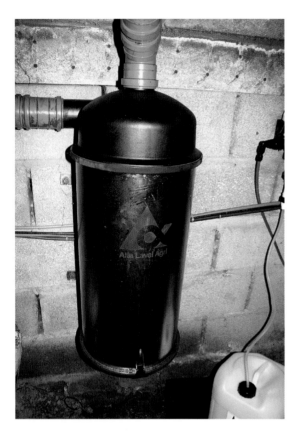

Interceptor vessel – prevents foreign material or liquid damaging the vacuum pump.

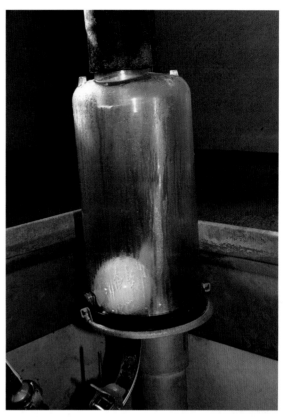

Sanitary trap – a ball valve between the milk and the air systems to prevent contamination of liquid into the air system.

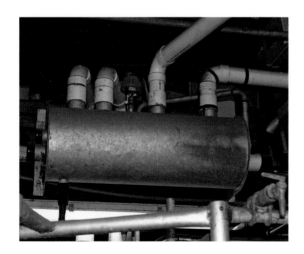

Balance tank – acts as a storage tank balancing and effectively increasing the plant's reserve.

Vacuum Gauge

A pressure gauge to indicate the level of the vacuum in the system by comparing atmospheric pressure with the partial vacuum within the plant. This can vary between 38kPa for a direct to line low line system to up to 50kPa for a recorder jar parlour.

Recorder Jar

A vessel to receive and hold all the milk from an individual animal, allowing yield measurement. Only present in non-direct to line systems and is situated between the long milk tube and the milk transfer line.

Receiver Vessel

In pipeline milking installations it is necessary to include a method of extracting the milk

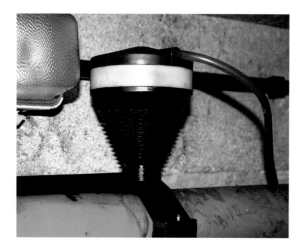

Regulator – an automatic valve to maintain a steady vacuum by allowing air to leak into the system. It should be 'hissing' all the time.

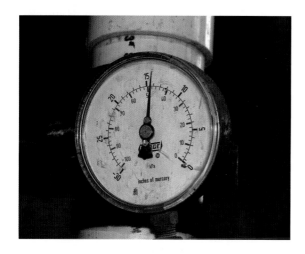

Vacuum gauge – pressure gauge indicating the level of vacuum in the plant compared to the atmospheric pressure.

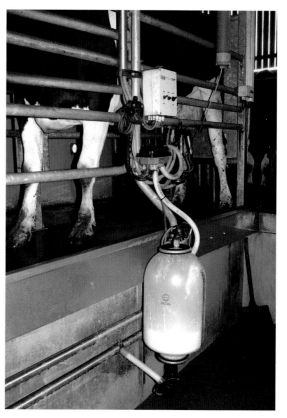

Recorder jar – a vessel, generally a glass jar, to hold milk from an individual cow. Not present in direct to line systems.

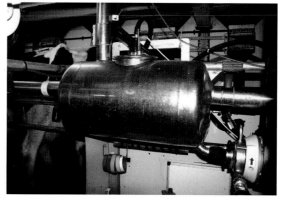

Receiver vessel – facilitates extraction of milk from the vacuum system to atmospheric pressure and to the bulk tank.

to an open storage bulk tank at atmospheric pressure from the vacuum system without the loss of vacuum. A receiver vessel receives milk from one or more milking transfer pipelines under vacuum and acts as a milk reservoir and air separator and then, during milking, the weight (activating a switch in older parlours) or level of milk (by an electrical probe in more modern parlours) in the receiver is used to start the milk pump which then transfers the milk to the bulk tank. It is generally constructed of either glass or, in more modern parlours, stainless steel which is more resistant to breakage but harder to inspect.

Milk Pump

A pressure pump to deliver milk along the delivery pipe from the receiver to the bulk milk tank.

Pipelines

- Main vacuum line: between the vacuum pump and the sanitary trap.
- Milk line: between the sanitary trap and the long milk tubes.
- Pulsation line: between the main vacuum line and the pulsator.
- Long milk tube: between the milk line and the clawpiece.
- Long pulsation tube: between the pulsator and the clawpiece.

Pulsators

A device that cyclically opens and closes the liner by alternating vacuum and atmospheric air within the pulsation chamber which is responsible for the milking process. The opening of the liner relies on the important inherent elasticity of the rubber when there

is no pressure difference across the inside and the outside of the liner.

Cluster

The cluster consists of a clawpiece and four teatcups containing the liners enclosed in hard shells which protect and support the liners. The liners and shells are connected to the clawpiece by a short milk tube and a short pulsation tube. The clawpiece itself is, in turn, connected to the long milk tube and the long pulsation tube.

Clawpiece or Claw

The clawpiece connects the four short milk tubes to the long milk tube via a milk reservoir called the bowl, while at the same time connecting the short pulsation tubes to the long pulsation tube. This arrangement facilitates

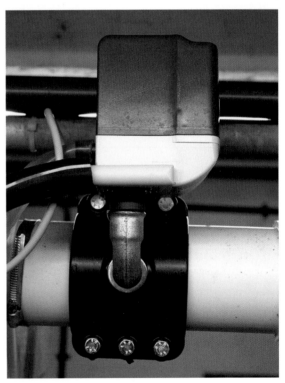

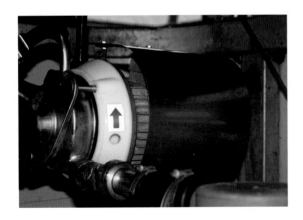

Milk pump – positive pressure pump to move milk along the delivery pipe to the bulk tank; works intermittently when receiver jar triggers the pump.

Pulsator – device to open and close the liner cyclically by alternating vacuum and atmosphere in the pulsation chamber within the shell.

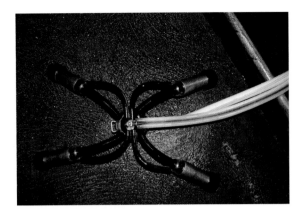

Cluster – consists of the clawpiece, four teatcups containing the liners enclosed in hard shells.

the intermittent flow of milk from each quarter along the long milk tube, made possible by the liner movements under the influence of cyclical vacuum fluctuations within the pulsation chamber. There is an airbleed hole in the clawpiece to aid the flow of milk from the bowl along the long milk tube. The volume of the bowl needs to be sufficient to prevent milk build-up, which would cause flooding and interfere with

the vacuum stability, particularly at the critical site of the teat end. Flooding would allow milk from one quarter to bathe the ends of the other teats, increasing the chance of cross-contamination and new intramammary infections, particularly when coupled with the associated vacuum fluctuations, causing a retrograde flow of milk and the impacts of this milk on the teat end. Clawpiece sizes were initially as little as 50ml but now, with high-yielding cows with high peak milk-flow rates, volumes have been increased to as much as 500ml; *see* diagram below.

Liners

Liners are the only component of the milking machine which come into contact with the cow; they consist of a mouthpiece, barrel and generally an integral short milk tube to connect it to the clawpiece. Liners have a limited working life, with most manufacturers quoting 2,500 milkings when they are made of the most commonly used material of synthetic compound rubber, although some are silicone-based, which extends their life to up to 10,000

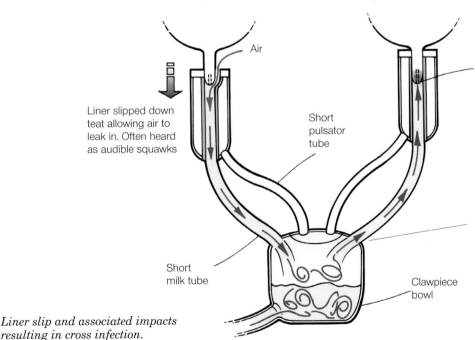

Liner slip and associated impacts resulting in cross infection.

Air

Liner slipped down teat allowing air to leak in. Often heard as audible squawks

Short milk tube

Short pulsator tube

Impact in teat end causing potential contamination and penetration of the streak canal by infected milk

Cross infection can also occur if milk flow from all four quarters into the clawpiece bowl overcomes the reservoir capacity of the clawpiece bowl and the ability of the vacuum to remove the milk before it floods up the short milk tubes and bathes the teat ends in potentially infected milk

Clawpiece bowl

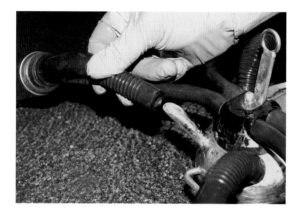

Clawpiece – connects the four short milk tubes to the long milk tube via the reservoir called the clawpiece bowl.

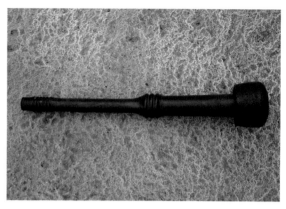

Liner – the only part of the milking machine in contact with the cow.

milkings. This life expectancy will be influenced by the numbers of cows being milked and the numbers of milking units available, as well as the number of wash-up routines (numbers of completed milkings) as the chemicals used in plant cleaning have an adverse effect on the liner surface. When a liner surface becomes rough and worn this can cause abrasions to the teat skin during milking, as well as being more difficult to clean and more likely to harbour bacteria (*see* liner replacement calculator spreadsheet under Further Reading). Research shows that measurable changes in liner elasticity are detectable, but not significant at as few as 1,000 milkings but do not affect performance until 2,500 milkings. This loss of elasticity changes the crispness of both liner opening, slowing milking down, and closing which can result in 'liner slap', where the saggy liner impacts the teat rather than smoothly squeezing it. This is confirmed by the fact that when particularly worn liners are replaced there is often a reduction in milking time.

Liner choice is critical to ensure minimal trauma to the cow's teats. They must have a soft, pliable mouthpiece to ensure an airtight seal with the teat base and reduce the chance of air incursions and liner slips or, in the extreme case, unit fall off. They must be compatible with the shells being used, the cow's teat size and teat length to ensure that the liner can

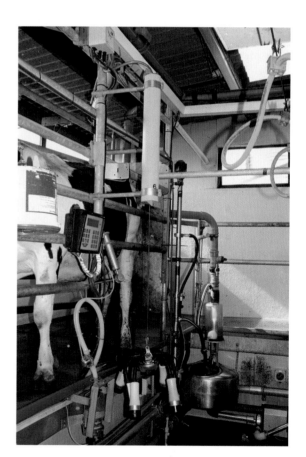

ACR or automatic cluster remover – shuts off the vacuum once the milk flow has dropped below a preset trigger point and a piston removes the cluster.

collapse below the teat end, giving a good rest or massage phase. Some liners are modified to try to reduce the chance of cross infection by reducing the chance of milk from one quarter coming into contact with that of other quarters during milking. Shielded liners, as their name suggests, have a perforated shield at the junction between the barrel and the short milk tube, reducing the chance of direct impacts of potentially infected milk on the teat end during retrograde flow during vacuum fluctuations. Ball valve liners attempt to take things further and overcome milk welling up and bathing the teat end in potentially infected milk, if flooding occurs.

Developments in liner design include the introduction of triangular shaped liners (rather than the normal round profile) and more recently these triangular liners have incorporated an air bleed at each liner mouthpiece as opposed to the more conventional single air bleed in the claw.

Automatic Cluster Remover (ACR)

ACRs remove the cluster automatically by shutting off the vacuum to the long milk tube when the milk flow has dropped below a preset trigger point. There is a delay from the trigger point to allow the vacuum to drop by air leaking in through the clawpiece airbleed before the unit is removed. There is a trend to 'wetter' milking, with trigger points being set at higher flow rates and the use of shorter delay times. This tends to leave higher strip yields but does not reduce total milk yields. *See* unit removal in milking routine.

Milk Filters

Bulk Milk Filter

While every attempt is made to avoid gross contamination of the milk supply, it is still possible for contamination from the surface of the udder, such as hair, earth, dung, bedding or milk clots not from the surface of the udder, to gain entry. It is also possible that contamination can be 'sucked' up if units fall off or are kicked off (*see* photo on page 132). Milk filters

are generally either single-use, material sock filters placed over the end of the delivery pipe, which are replaced each milking, or an in-line cartridge filter of pierced nylon plastic or stainless steel screens usually of two gauges (coarse 150 and fine 75 microns) which are rinsed and washed in disinfectant after each milking. Often two sets are used so that one is soaking in disinfectant while the other is in use. Filters are unable to remove particles smaller than 70 microns or they become clogged with milk fat.

Individual Cow Filters for Detecting Mastitis

In-line filters in the long milk tube can be an aid to mastitis detection but they need to be checked after every cow has been milked so mastitic cows can be identified. They also act as a coarse filter removing extraneous material.

Delivery Pipeline

A pipeline carrying milk under positive pressure from the milk pump to the bulk tank often via a plate cooler.

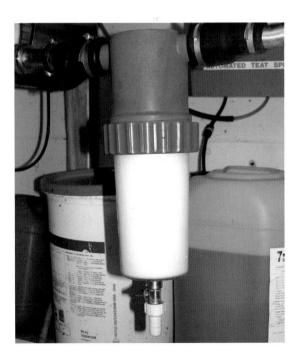

Bulk tank filter in situ *during milking.*

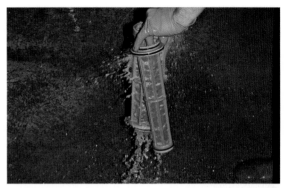

Bulk tank filter removed.

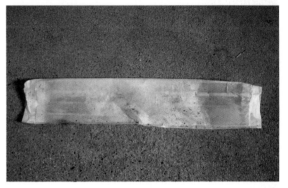

Bulk tank filter being rinsed before being immersed in disinfectant.

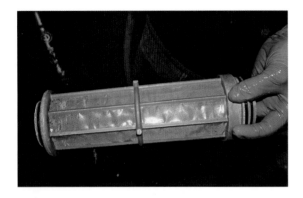

Bulk tank filter separated.

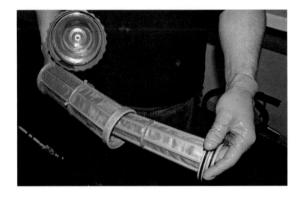

Bulk tank sock, showing faecal contamination.

Plate Cooler

A heat exchange system where the cooling effect of water circulated through the plate cooler is used to improve the efficiency and speed of milk cooling while also reducing energy (electricity) costs.

Bulk Tank

On farm refrigerated bulk storage for milk awaiting collection.

Milk Tanker

Refrigerated lorry to collect farm milk and deliver it to the dairy to be processed.

Vacuum Pump Capacity

The air moving capability of the pump (ltr/min) can be assessed as follows:

Working Vacuum

Stabilized vacuum level with liners plugged and accessories connected but not operating.

Effective Reserve

Vacuum pump effective reserve capacity is measured with the regulator *working* and then admitting air near the regulator to lower the pressure 2.0kPa below the working vacuum.

Manual Reserve

Vacuum pump manual reserve capacity is measured with the regulator *inactivated* and then admitting air near the regulator to lower the pressure 2.0kPa below the working vacuum.

Pulsation

Pulsation is the movement of the liner around the teat from open to closed.

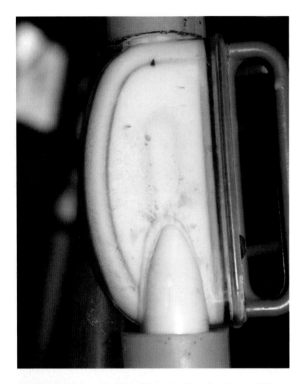

Individual cow in-line filter in situ *during milking.*

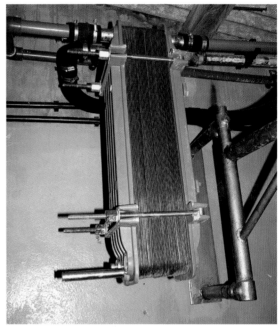

Plate cooler – cold water is circulated through the plate cooler to aid milk cooling.

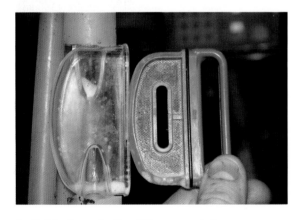

Individual cow in-line filter separated.

Open or Milking Phase
While the liner is open, a vacuum is applied at the teat end and milk is removed by a pressure differential.

Closed Massage or Rest Phase
The pulsator admits atmospheric air to the pulsation chamber between the liner and the shell. This collapses the liner on the teat and provides massage to it. This alternate cycle of liner open milking phase and liner closed massage phase is necessary because, while the milk is removed during the milking phase by vacuum, the vacuum also draws blood and body fluids down into the teat. Without adequate massage the teat and the teat end may become engorged and oedematous causing damage and increasing the risk of mastitis.

Pulsation Rate
The number of pulsation cycles per minute. Most parlours are set in a range of 50 to 60 cycles per minute.

Simultaneous Pulsation: '4 and nothing'
The cyclic movement of all liners within a cluster is synchronized.

Alternate Pulsation: '2 and 2'
The cyclic movement of half the number of liners within a cluster alternates with the

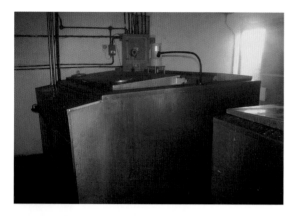

Bulk tank – older ice jacket type.

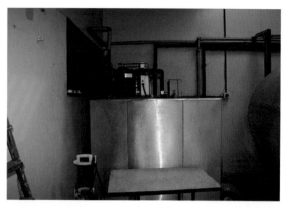

Bulk tank ice bank.

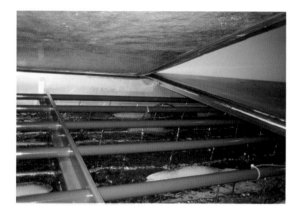

Bulk tank ice bank with lid raised to show ice production.

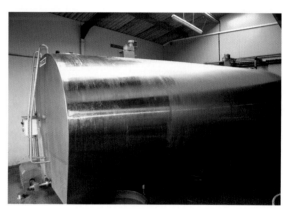

Bulk tank – large, modern, bulk tank.

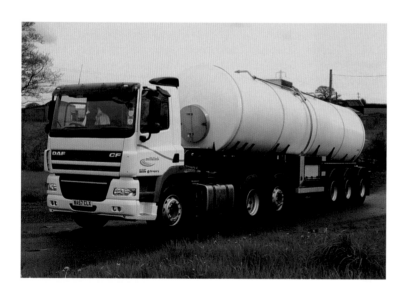

Milk tanker – milk is collected from the farm by a refrigerated lorry.

movement of the other half. With alternate pulsation there is a possibility for an unintentional difference between the two pulsator ratios of, say, 62:38 and 58:42, giving a difference of 4 per cent which is termed 'limping'. It is generally thought that the magnitude of this difference should be kept to less than 2 to 3 per cent.

Pulsation Ratio

The setting or ratio of the open milking phase and the closed or massage phase is critical and this makes the pulsator very important in the milking process. If the milking phases are too short, quarters will not be milked out effectively or may milk out very slowly. If the massage phase does not take place or is too short, oedema of the teat will occur and the quarter will not be milked properly. On top of this, teat end damage will occur. Either situation is bad for udder health.

The pulsation ratio is the proportion of one pulsation cycle that the milking machine is in the milking phase compared to the massage phase. Most common ratios are between 50:50 and 70:30, with perhaps 60:40 being the most common. In theory, in low line installations vacuum levels can be dropped and pulsation ratios widened to a higher ratio, resulting in faster milking with lower unit-on times. This is the one time where both milker and cow benefit from faster milking. Lower unit-on time means fewer squeezes to the teat end for each cow milked and the milker will milk more cows per hour and get home quicker.

Pulsation Cycle within the Pulsation Chamber

The pressure changes within the pulsation chamber are an indirect measure of the liner wall movements and can be measured to give a graphical print-out (trace) of the current pulsation rate and ratio. One complete pulsation cycle, where the liner opens and then closes, can be divided into four phases a, b, c and d.

The pulsation ratio is defined as the ratio between the milking phase and the resting (massage) phase and is generally never more than 50 per cent massage phase. Consequently, 'wide' pulsation ratios have longer milking phases than massage phase, for example, 60:40 or, more extreme, 70:30.

$$\text{Pulsation ratio} = \frac{a + b}{c + d} \times 100\%$$

Problems Associated with Variations in the Pulsation Trace

As the b phase is 'active' and created by the application of a vacuum to the pulsation chamber, it rarely exceeds the manufacturer's specification. The c phase, however, can be a useful indicator of the most common problems, other than incorrect set-up, with in general shorter c phases being associated with air leaks.

A shortened c phase (rapid aggressive closing) may result from air leaks into the pulsation chamber from cracks or splits in the long or the short pulse tubing, especially if combined with a lengthened a phase (slow delayed opening); air is leaking into the pulsation chamber accentuating closure and delaying the opening of the liner.

A lengthened c phase (slow delayed closing), often with a normal a phase and possibly

Phases of one complete pulsation cycle

Phase	Liner activity	Effect	Phase
a	Liner opening	Milk flow initiates	Milking
b	Liner open	Maximum milk flow	Milking
c	Liner closing	Milk flow reducing	Resting (Massage)
d	Liner closed	No milk flow – teat massage and blood circulates	Resting (Massage)

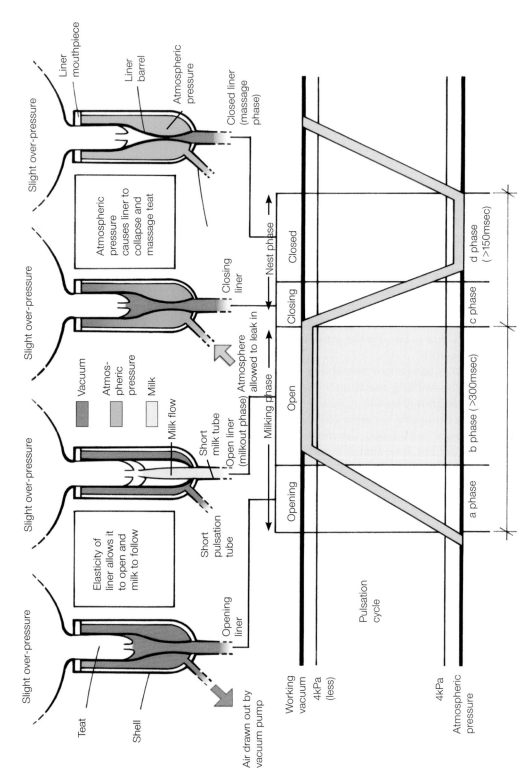

Comparison of pressure changes within the pulsation chamber represented on a graphical trace and the movement of the liner within the shell during the pulsation cycle.

shortened d phase (reduced massage time), may indicate restricted air flow to the pulsator from a blocked air port or filter; air is slowly admitted to the pulsation chamber, delaying closure and reducing the effectiveness of teat massage; this might also result in variation in the d phase.

Variation in the d phase vacuum level may indicate that the pulsator is unable to maintain liner closure because of insufficient air being admitted to the pulsation chamber due to a blocked pulsator filter.

An incomplete d phase (liner does not fully close), where the trace does not reach atmospheric pressure, although the trace may be horizontal, indicates that the pulsator valve is not closing properly and may be dirty; some air continues to be removed from the pulsation chamber preventing full liner closure.

A lengthened a phase (slow opening) and lengthened c phase (slow closing) indicate restricted air flow in both directions and might indicate kinked or restricted pulsation tubes, that the diameter may be too small or the length too long; inefficient air movement in the pulsation system reduces the crispness of liner opening and closing.

Routine and Regular Maintenance and Testing

Daily Checks
Many checks may well be done automatically by the milker who is using the machine, such as ensuring that the vacuum gauge shows correct vacuum, the regulator is 'hissing' and the pulsators sound right. Visual inspection of rubberwork for cracks or splits, along with checking that the air bleed is not blocked are also important. The milker may be suspicious that something is wrong by noticing a change in machine function such as increased milking time or units falling off for no apparent reason.

Monthly or Weekly Checks
Checking the cleanliness of air filters in the regulator and pulsators will ensure that they are not clogged with dust or dirt. The vacuum pump oil level and belt tension need checking to ensure that it will function efficiently. The sanitary trap should be checked for moisture.

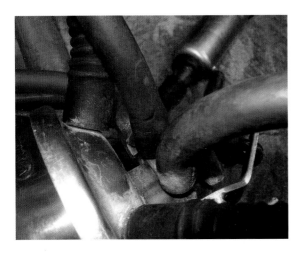

Split, short pulsation tube which will tend to result in aggressive liner closure and delay in the opening of the liner.

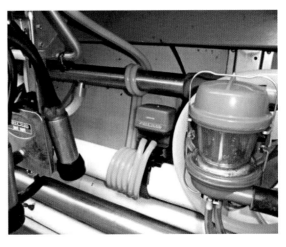

This unusual set-up will restrict air flow and result in the slow opening and closing of the liners.

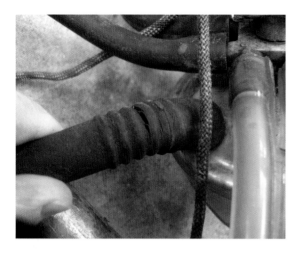

Split, short milk tube.

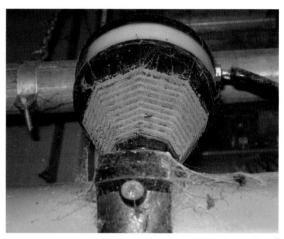

Dirty vacuum regulator.

Routine Milking Machine Tests Usually Performed by a Specialist Milking Machine Technician

Static

A test to check that the milking machine is functioning correctly and that the settings are within British Standards and the manufacturer's specifications under non-milking conditions. Vacuum pump capacity, vacuum level, vacuum reserve, pulsation rate and ratio are all checked, along with a thorough visual inspection of the rubberwork. Liner condition and liner replacement intervals should be checked and compared with the manufacturer's recommendations (generally 2,500 milkings).

Dynamic

Unlike a static test the dynamic test checks vacuum levels and fluctuations close to the teat end of a few cows while they are being milked. Generally, high-yielding cows are used as this will emphasize any inadequacies in the parlour function. The traces from the test equipment are used to observe vacuum levels and stability, milk flows, ACR take-off settings (switch point and delay), as well as taking note of cow behaviour and post-milking teat condition. Liner slips both audible and those identified by the traces are recorded and strip yields

may be checked to measure the completeness of milking.

Vacuum Fluctuations

The fluctuations in the vacuum in the liner have important effects on milk flow, encouraging retrograde flow which can have a significant influence on mastitis rates.

There are two types of vacuum fluctuation:

1. **Irregular** These occur when the liners slip or fall from the teats or when air enters when the milking units are changed carelessly; vacuum recovery will be slow if there is insufficient vacuum reserve.
2. **Cyclic (regular)** The cyclic movements of the liner in each pulsation cycle increase and decrease the volume of the liner under the teat; when milk is flowing this can cause marked changes in the vacuum below the teat and these cyclical fluctuations can be reduced by using wide-bore short milk tubes (>8mm) and ensuring that claw air bleeds are not blocked.

Simple Investigation

Many simple observations, such as a drop in the vacuum when units are opened to check vacuum reserve or the insertion of a thumb in the liners to check pulsation rate and liner

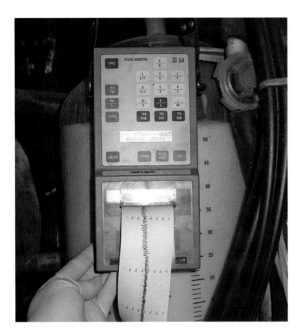

Alphatronic dynamic milking machine tester.

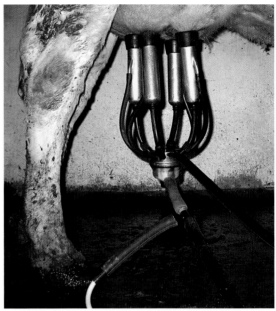

Alphatronic dynamic milking machine tester in use.

closure can be useful quick checks for milking-machine problems.

HYGIENE AND EFFECTIVE PLANT CLEANING

Much has been written on milking-machine cleaning and it is beyond the scope of this book to be a reference text. The basic concepts of the two most common wash-up routines, circulation and acid boiling wash, are detailed. When cleaning anything water is generally an essential part. However, additional components often play a part in augmenting the cleaning process and cleaning a milking machine is no different. Often when cleaning an object hot water is used (thermal energy), chemicals are added to the cleaning solution (chemical energy) and scrubbing, or, in the case of a parlour, air injectors produce an agitation of the circulating water often causing the parlour to shake (mechanical energy) to help to improve the cleaning process. Although increasing the time of the action of cleaning can often also improve the process, this is not the case with milking-machine cleaning.

There is an optimal time for circulating the hot chemical solution after which, if it is continued, the results deteriorate.

If there are problems with the wash-up routine both milk residues and bacteria are likely to build up within the plant and bactoscan will increase and can result in financial penalties to the producer. Clearly all parts of the plant need to be cleaned and, consequently, an adequate volume, temperature and chemical concentration are required. The units are mounted in the upright position on a rack of teat-cup jetters which are connected to the washline which swirl the circulating cleaner around the liner and complete the circuit.

Circulation Cleaning

Although automatic systems are becoming more common, even they need some human intervention such as washing the outsides of the units and attaching them to the jetters; the vast majority of parlour wash up routines require some form of human intervention. This also includes the amounts of hot and cold water introduced by the movement of the suction and return pipes, followed by the

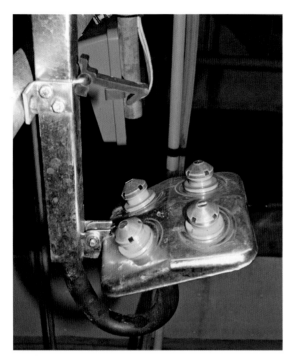

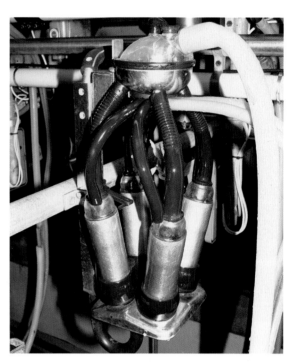

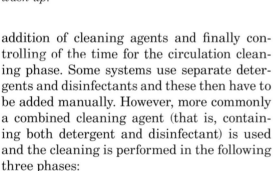

Jetters – facilitate cleaning of the clusters during wash-up.

Liners on jetters.

addition of cleaning agents and finally controlling of the time for the circulation cleaning phase. Some systems use separate detergents and disinfectants and these then have to be added manually. However, more commonly a combined cleaning agent (that is, containing both detergent and disinfectant) is used and the cleaning is performed in the following three phases:

Rinse
A pre-rinse, usually with lukewarm water, to get rid of most of the milk residues after milking. The rinse should continue until the discarded effluent water is clear.

Wash and Disinfection
Circulation cleaning with a cleaning solution containing a combined detergent and disinfectant agent. The water temperature should be between 70° and 90°C (160° to 190°F) when it is introduced, falling to between 40° and 50°C (105° to 120°F) at the end of the circulation. The

end temperature should never be below 40°C since this could cause the formation of fatty coatings. Air is often admitted to the system to encourage 'slug' flow with some associated turbulence to aid cleaning. Air injectors are often used in large-bore milking parlours to facilitate this.

Final Rinse
A final rinse, usually with cold water, to remove any residues of the cleaning solution.

In systems using detergents and disinfectants separately two further phases will be performed. After the detergent cleaning, the plant is rinsed and then a disinfection circulation follows. After the disinfection, a final rinse will usually be performed.

Acid Boiling Wash (ABW)
Despite ABW being simpler than circulation cleaning, it is not very popular in the United Kingdom. It relies entirely on the chemicals and heat to clean the parlour, without any

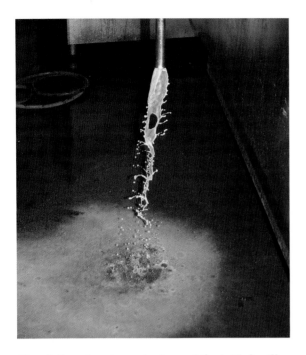

Circulation cleaning – rinsing out the initial milk residues.

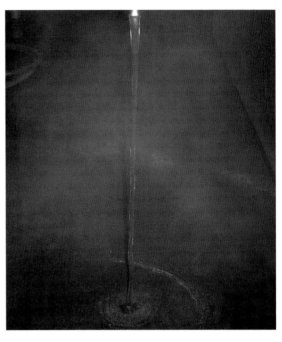

Circulation cleaning – once the flow becomes clear, circulation can be started.

recirculation. Large volumes of boiling water are needed, which take the same route as circulation cleaning but are run around the plant direct to waste. ABW is faster than circulation cleaning, uses smaller amounts of chemicals but requires larger volumes of hot water.

Milkstone Removal

In particularly hard water areas minerals can accumulate as deposits within the pipework of the parlour. This can be seen as a chalky film and is generally formed by the cations of calcium, magnesium and iron. Phosphoric acid solutions

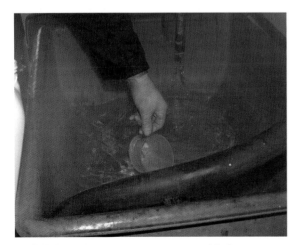

Circulation cleaning – chemical is added once circulation has been initiated.

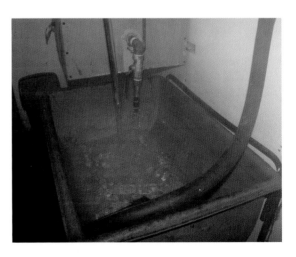

Circulation cleaning – circulation.

are effective as milkstone removers and are commonly run through a parlour as required.

MILKING ROUTINE AND ITS IMPORTANCE IN MASTITIS CONTROL

The National Mastitis Council's (NMC) recommended milking procedures include these steps as part of a complete routine:

1. Provide a clean, low-stress environment for cows.
2. Check foremilk and udder for mastitis.
3. Wash teats with an udder wash solution or pre-dip teats in an effective product.
4. Dry teats completely with an individual towel.
5. Attach milking unit within 2min of the start of stimulation.
6. Adjust units as necessary for proper alignment.
7. Shut off vacuum before removing unit.
8. Dip teats immediately after unit removal with an effective product.

1. GENERAL CONCEPTS

Milk is produced throughout the day by the secretory tissue (alveoli) deep within the udder. Much of the milk is also stored within these alveoli and small ducts with the remainder of the milk being stored in the larger ducts and udder cistern (cisternal milk). In order for milk to be removed from the udder, either by a milking machine or by a suckling calf, the cow needs to be stimulated to 'let her milk down' in response to oxytocin released from the pituitary gland in the brain into the blood by both tactile stimuli, of predominantly the sensitive receptors in the teat skin, as well as by psychological stimuli such as sights and sounds. As a result of this, avoiding cows becoming stressed or frightened before or during milking as well as ensuring a consistency of milking routine is essential for effective milk let-down. Incomplete milk let-down will increase the milking time for each

cow, resulting in more trauma to the teat end as more pulsation phases will occur (opening and closing of the liner), which will often result in increased mastitis. Optimum times for stimulation before the unit is attached and milk flow is initiated are generally recognized to be between 1 and 2min. Any longer than this and the oxytocin concentrations in the blood drop rapidly and milk let-down is reduced. Teat preparation (often quoted as being optimally 20sec to maximize oxytocin release and achieve effective cleaning) needs to be fitted into this routine.

Preparation for the Milkers

General Hygiene

Cleanliness within the parlour itself is important for the production of high quality milk, as is operator cleanliness such as washing hands and changing into clean milking clothes. Milkers should wear specially assigned, waterproof clothing. This might be leggings and a parlour top or an apron or sometimes waterproof sleeves. The spread of infection within the milking parlour can be via three main routes: the milker's hands, the use of cloths or towels and the milking machine itself, and generally the liner.

Gloves

The wearing of gloves by milkers can greatly reduce the chance of the spread of mastitis pathogens in the parlour. This is not by any unexplained, magical properties of gloves, but will, in part, be due to the fact that human skin, particularly hands used to manual work, can harbour bacteria able to cause mastitis in cattle (most notably *Staphylococcus aureus*) and act as source of infection, and, in part, that gloves are easy to disinfect, which helps to reduce the fomite route of spreading of infections within the parlour.

Repeated hand washing can adversely affect the condition of the milkers' hands and so milkers wearing gloves tend to wash their hands more frequently during milking, which also helps to improve milk hygiene as well as reducing the chance of spreading mastitis pathogens during milking. The adoption and long-term compliance of milkers wearing gloves is greatly influenced by the type of glove chosen. Non-disposable gloves tend to be quite thick and can make milking arduous. Nitrile gloves are often green, purple or blue and are generally more comfortable and robust than white 'dental' latex gloves, which often have powder or latex proteins inside them which can be an irritant to the milkers' hands. Although cheap, the white 'dental' gloves are very thin and tend to break easily, often resulting in just a white cuff around the wrist. Gloves used for milking should be disposed of at the end of milking and, in larger herds, they may need to be replaced during milking as well.

Preparation of the Cow

2. MASTITIS DETECTION RATHER THAN DIAGNOSIS

'Cow-side' Detection – Now and in the Future

In its simplest form mastitis detection will be the observation of changes in one or any combination of the following: the visible appearance of the milk, the udder either visually or palpably (or both) and perhaps a change in the cow's demeanour. Some of these changes may be obvious even to the unskilled eye, while others may be more subtle and require not only husbandry skills and experience but also knowledge of the normal udder shape and fullness, as well as the usual behaviour of that individual cow. Cows are very much creatures of habit and are comforted by a routine. Equally, they will often add to the consistency of the routine by entering the parlour in a similar order each time they are milked. Clues that a cow is suffering from a case of mastitis might include being more fidgety than normal while being prepared for milking or entering the parlour to be milked out of her normal sequence in the herd. For example, a mastitic cow that is normally early into the parlour to be milked may be not feeling too well and as a result may be out of her normal sequence and be milked nearer the

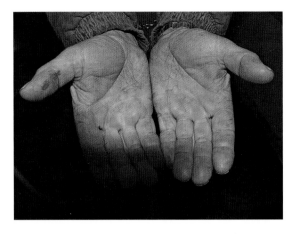

Hands are difficult to clean and often have cracks which harbour bacteria.

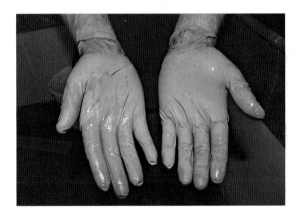

New gloves – no more than one milking per set of gloves and they may need to be replaced during milking.

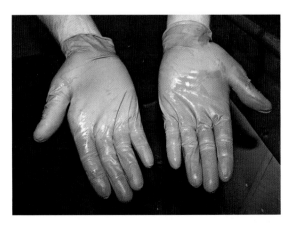

Used gloves.

end of milking. The observation approach discussed above is expanded beyond what is essentially good husbandry and looking after animal welfare to encompass food safety, so that when cows are being milked to produce milk for human consumption, no abnormal milk is allowed to enter the human food chain.

Legal Requirements

It is stated within the Dairy Products (Hygiene) Regulations 1995 that 'at the start of the milking of an individual animal, the milker shall inspect the appearance of the milk' and that contaminated milk 'shall not be allowed to leave the production holding'. It is therefore the farmer's responsibility to take appropriate action to check milk quality by examination for the presence of blood, clots and discoloration.

Methods of inspecting the milk include:

- foremilking
- conductivity meter/colour detection system
- transparent clusters
- long milk tube filters
- recording jars.

The inspecting of the appearance of the milk can be routine and active as in foremilking, automated in in-line detection with a parlour warning system or it can be by visual observation which may or may not be performed, such as inspecting long milk tube filters or observing the recorder jar milk.

Foremilking

If performed as part of the milking routine this gives a consistent and regular check for mastitis prior to each cow being milked. Foremilking is best performed *before* teat preparation, providing that the teats are fairly clean, and involves removing a few (four or five) squirts of milk by hand. This way mastitis-causing bacteria transmitted by the action of foremilking can be eliminated by pre-milking sanitation. If the teats are not clean when the cows come into the parlour foremilking can be done after washing, provided that they are sanitized again before the units are attached. There are a number of benefits other than early detection of mastitis. The action of handling the teats should act as a stimulus to aid milk let-down and, as the foremilk contains high bacterial counts, this may contribute towards reducing mastitis risk.

Visual Observation

There are also potential visual observations that can be made during the milking process, but there is no assurance that they will be performed for each cow. These would include observation of the udder for signs of swelling or discoloration, observation of the recorder jar or transparent cluster and checking the in-line long milk tube filter. Recorder jar and transparent cluster observation are at least specific to the particular cow being milked (provided in the case of recorder jar observation that all the milk is transferred after each cow is milked). The in-line, long milk tube filter, however, can be left unobserved for several cows, if not the whole milking, in which case it will not be apparent which cow has clots in its milk. In a similar fashion, if mastitis detection is poor the milk sock or bulk filter can sometimes be observed having clots in it.

Automated In-line

Automated systems happen routinely. Their ability to detect mastitis relies on comparison with previous readings giving within-cow comparison and comparison over time. These systems are essential in automatic milking systems (AMS), sometimes known as robotic milking. There is no routine human presence or intervention with AMS and so a system is needed to both detect mastitis and protect the human food chain. Electroconductivity is perhaps the most commonly employed automated measurement used to trigger an 'alarm' for mastitis. Milk yield and colour have also been used and there is a potential for in-line systems for SCC using CMT, lactate dehydrogenase (LDH) and acute phase proteins (APP), notably milk amyloid A (MAA) to be used for early detection in automated systems.

Detection or Diagnosis?

There are a number of tests that are effectively detection tests but are often used in such a way that they are, to all intents and purposes, confirmatory diagnostic tests. In this situation there would be a suspicion that a cow is suffering from a case of mastitis and these tests would be used to identify whether that is the case and which quarters (or quarter) are affected, with a view to either monitoring, treating or subjecting the milk to bacteriological culture. Under these circumstances the tests are being used to confirm a diagnosis of mastitis. Tests that are used in this way for SCC estimations would include: the California Milk Test (CMT), hand-held electroconductivity meters and the Delaval Direct Cell Counter. Other indicators of udder health, such as cellular ATP using Lacdetect photometer or acute phase protein estimation, for example, MAA, can also be used as confirmatory diagnostic tests in this way.

CMT

CMT is a mastitis test which is very much a cow-side test and can be done in real time (taking a few seconds), but, despite being very cheap and easy to perform, it is still fiddly enough not to be used as a screening test on a regular basis. The CMT gives an estimate of SCC by the reagent, a detergent, denaturing the DNA in the somatic cells (and, to a certain extent, any bacteria present). giving a slimy gel reaction. Many CMT kits also have a pH indicator, bromcresol purple, which is sensitive and changes to a dark purple colour in response to the increasing pH seen in mastitic milk. CMT has a limit of detection and, because of the dilution effect of, say, three clean quarters and one infected quarter resulting in a 'negative' SCC at a cow level, it is best performed at a quarter level. It can be used to screen quarters before drying off (say, a couple of times a week apart just before drying off) or after calving (optimally three

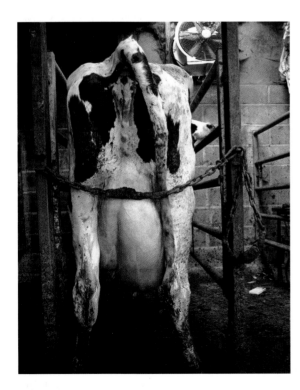

Swollen quarter.

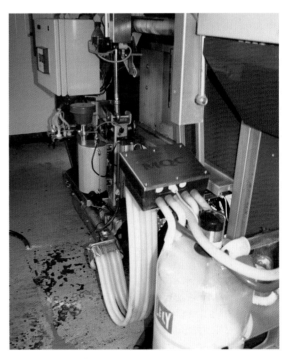

Robot or automatic milking system (AMS), 'Automatic milk conductivity' (AMC) in-line electroconductivity.

to five days after calving) to estimate infection status (particularly useful in first lactation heifers), as well as being used to confirm suspicions that a cow has mastitis. Equally, CMT can also be used to monitor quarters in cows known to be infected, either to check for a cure if treatment has been undertaken or to see whether self-cure has occurred. As CMT is cheap and easy to perform, it can be repeated frequently to monitor individual quarters in problem cows.

As a result of the threshold of SCC detection for CMT being quite close to the recognized cow infection threshold of 200,000 cells/ml but significantly above the increasingly recognized quarter infection threshold of 100,000 cells, it is important to use even a slight change (trace) to identify infected quarters. When a CMT value of 'trace' or greater is used, in excess of 90 per cent of infected cows will be correctly identified. However, if a CMT value of >1 is used, then fewer than 75 per cent of infected cows will be correctly identified. To minimize the number of false negative results, the test should be read as positive when at least a trace reaction is apparent.

Hand-held
Electroconductivty (EC) Meter
Hand-held EC meters are available in many different countries (*see* photo on page 100). Their diagnostic accuracy is somewhat variable and independent work has shown that 71 per cent of the test-positive samples were bacteriologically negative and that major mastitis bacteria were isolated from 11 per cent of the test-negative samples. When used on individual quarters other screening tests such as CMT and individual SCCs appear to be more useful than hand-held EC meters. However, when a comparison of EC values between the quarters of the cow is used, this does help to reduce the intrinsic variation. Other daily and cow-specific variations also occur and in AMS, where EC is often the only detection method currently available, computer analysis of EC data is used to compare both between quarters and over time.

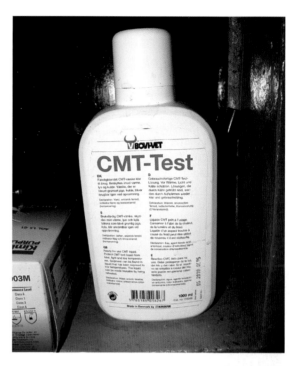

CMT container.

Delaval Direct Cell Counter (DCC)
The Delaval Direct Cell Counter (DCC) is a new device designed to be used on farms for rapid SCC evaluation. Small cassettes are filled with approximately 1 microlitre of fresh milk, stained automatically in the cassette and inserted into a small battery-operated optical cell counter. The DCC produces an SCC in less than 1min within the range of 10,000 to 4,000,000 cells/ml and with similar accuracy to monthly milk recording.

Future Developments
Detection rather than diagnosis has less significant constraints and targets for future developments but nonetheless still has many hurdles to overcome before the accomplishment of the ultimate goal of an automated, accurate, rapid (in line) and non-invasive reliable detection method is reached. Currently observation of the milk itself, by various methods ranging from the naked eye to electroconductivity, is the most common and accurate method giving swift and reasonably accurate early mastitis

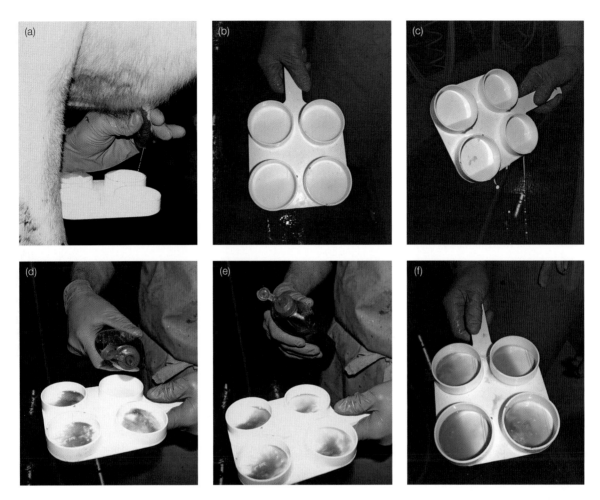

(a) CMT – collecting milk from each quarter. (b) Milk in each well from individual quarters. (c) Surplus milk tipped away down to a ridge in each well. (d) Reagent added and reaction often seen immediately. (e) Paddle is agitated to mix the milk and reagent. (f) Final result.

detection. Other measurement methodologies for udder inflammation are constantly being investigated, developed and evaluated with them all giving some indication of udder health with variable correlation to SCC.

Milk Amyloid A (MAA)

The severity of clinical signs of mastitis caused by a number of bacteria has been shown to correlate well with the concentration of a number of acute phase proteins in milk including amyloid A. Work has also been done comparing MAA and the more commonly measured cellular response such as SCC. MAA results

correlate reasonably well with SCC and may have an advantage in late lactation by not being affected by non-inflammatory changes within the udder, unlike SCC where increases can be as a result of reduced yield and dilution coupled with physiological changes within the udder. Some work has also indicated that MAA can give an indication of the causative bacteria, making it closer to diagnosis and not just detection.

Lacdetect Cellular ATP Measurement

Lacdetect is a test under development where a milk sample, either as a commingled cow

Grading CMT reactions: defining CMT scores and estimates of corresponding SCC

CMT score	Description	Est. SCC (cells/ml)	Interpretation
(Negative)	Mixture remains free-running liquid with no evidence of thickening or formation of a precipitate despite continued rotation of the paddle	<200,000	No mastitis
T (Trace)	Slight thickening that tends to disappear with continued rotation of the paddle	200,000 to 500,000	Suspicious
1 (Weak) +	Significant thickening, but little or no tendency toward gel formation. Thickening may disappear after prolonged rotation of the paddle	400,000 to 1,500,000	Suspicious
2 (Distinct) ++	Mixture thickens immediately. With continued rotation of the paddle, a gel accumulates in the centre of the well, leaving the outer edges exposed	800,000 to 5,000,000	Mastitis
3 (Strong) +++	A very obvious thick gel forms, which tends to stick to the bottom of the paddle forming a distinct lump in the centre of the well	Over 5,000,000	Mastitis

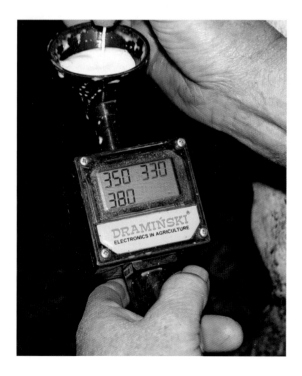

Hand-held electroconductivity tester.

sample from all four quarters or a quarter sample, is tested by using a dipstick in a small tube where cellular-derived ATP is measured by bioluminescence by using a photometer. It is hoped that this test will become a commercial, real-time, cow-side test giving results that closely correlate with SCC. It seems that this correlation with SCC may mean that parity and stage of lactation will have significant effects on milk ATP content similar to those on SCC.

Thermography

Technological advances through miniaturization, automation of data recording and the use of the computer analysis of data to pick up early trends may well mean that other parameters may show promise for the detection of mastitis. Some very preliminary work has been done using infra-red technology to measure the surface temperature of the udder as an early indicator of inflammation. Research is on-going and computer software will be needed to tease out the variation in udder surface temperature as a result of the udder inflammation from those of circadian (daily) fluctuations, temperature changes following exercise and, of course, the influence of the environmental factors such as temperature, moisture or even recent exposure to strong sunlight. The data show that the computer analysis (lag regression analysis) of previous daily udder temperatures, together with environmental temperature parameters, could successfully predict current udder temperature with a high degree of accuracy. So it is possible that at some time in the future infra-red thermography, if coupled with environmental temperature monitoring, could have a place as an early detection method for mastitis.

Automatic milking systems (AMS) robotic milking detection systems will, by definition, need to produce on-line automatic mastitis detection. Initially electroconductivity (EC) was the norm with sequential and inter-quarter readings within the same cow being compared by computer software to improve accuracy. However, many farmers found that the 'attention list' was often too long and false positives were a nuisance. Combining conductivity with yield data helps to improve accuracy.

In-line Automated CMT
Giving an SCC Estimation
More recently, on-line automated CMT has been introduced on some AMS installations. These are not only a cost to purchase the hardware, but each time the estimation of SCC is performed the reagents used for each quarter CMT test also have a cost implication. It seems that there may be a benefit to run an automated CMT after an EC alert rather than on every quarter at every milking. The test could be performed at the same milking by the EC alert triggering the AMS system to perform a CMT estimation on the milk. On-going research suggests that the combination of EC and CMT measures increases diagnostic accuracy severalfold.

LDH (Lactate Dehydrogenase)
Experimental work is on-going in looking for a cheap, fast mastitis indicator. LDH estimation on-line and in real time has advantages as it is very quick to perform but also incurs costs each time the test is run. Automatic real-time mastitis detection systems can be improved in both the sensitivity of detecting mastitis and the specificity of not giving a false positive diagnosis by the use of computer software. The software combines real-time LDH information with additional factors such as the number of days from calving, breed, parity, milk yield, udder characteristics, other disease records, electrical conductivity and herd characteristics. The output comprises a risk of acute mastitis and a relative degree of chronic mastitis. The software also produces a days-to-next sample value that allows sampling frequency to be either increased or reduced, depending on the risk of mastitis. It was able to detect mastitis reasonably well, with a sensitivity for detecting clinical mastitis of 82 per cent. Specificity, that is, the ability to avoid misclassifying healthy observations as mastitis, was 99 per cent.

There is much on-going research to find the best on-line, real-time indicator of clinical mastitis and, not surprisingly, no one parameter suffices. It seems that a combination of EC with confirmatory CMT and also using LDH and yield with significant software interpretation may be the route to the best results. This shows that, as is often the case, automating something a skilled manual worker does can be difficult.

3. TEAT PREPARATION

It has been known for many years that the new intramammary infection rate is related to the number of bacteria the teat end is exposed to. Further to this, much has been written about the relationship between clean housing and so clean cows and lower bulk tank SCC. By reducing the faecal contamination of the udder and, in particular, the teat end, mastitis rates from environmental bacteria such as coliforms

The Milking Machine and Milking Routine

and *Streptococcus uberis* can be significantly reduced. This overall and more holistic cleanliness in terms of presenting the cow in a clean state as she enters the parlour can be further enhanced by physical cleaning and disinfecting the teat prior to milking. As with any food production, hygiene is critical and unwanted bacterial contamination must be kept to a minimum. Equally, avoiding sediments such as soil or faeces in milk, which may occur if teats are muddy or contaminated with faeces, is important. Consequently, clean, sanitized teats have obvious advantages in milk quality. Higher sediment levels tend to be correlated with higher levels of environmental mastitis and increased TBC. Any improvements in teat cleanliness by teat preparation (cleaning and disinfection) just prior to the cows are milked will be reflected in improvements in milk quality, particularly in terms of bacterial load. As a consequence, the various measurements of milk hygiene such as total bacterial (viable) count TBC/TVC and bactoscan will be demonstrably improved where effective pre-milking teat sanitization is employed. Options used for pre-milking teat preparation are shown in the table below. The effectiveness, time taken and likely uptake by operators all vary. Clearly some methods are significantly better at sanitizing the teats than others.

The factors involved when considering the method of teat preparation to be employed in a herd will include cost, time involved (available labour), required effect (depending on initial teat cleanliness, BMSCC and bactoscan) and, more recently, issues of environmental impact. Significant amounts of paper towel are used in preparation for milking and the energy and resources for their production, as well as disposal impacts in terms of landfill, are making washing and drying of individual flannel towels more attractive. Economic studies have shown that cost effectiveness will even include the purchase of washing and drying

Options for teat preparation before milking

Method	Options
None	N/A
Dry wipe	Gloved hand or paper towel (ideally individual use). Can be combined with pre-dip afterwards
Antiseptic impregnated individual wipe	Formulated to evaporate and so no paper drying required. May require multiple dispensers depending on size of parlour to avoid excessive walking in parlour
Wash and dry	Drop lines and individual paper or flannel towel
Pre-dip and individual paper or flannel towel	Various products available including dips, sprays and gels. May require wash first especially if teats soiled
Mechanical driven rotating brushes	Semi-automatic – hand held. Automatic in AMS (robot milking). Disinfectant water sanitizes and brushes clean and then rotate rapidly to dry teat

machines, although some work shows that a hot detergent wash may remove the need for hot air drying. The clean flannel towels can be stored in a clean, dry dustbin with a tightly fitting lid. The same requirements for correct udder preparation procedures with paper towels apply when using flannel towels. A freshly laundered towel must be used for each cow at each milking. The entire teat, including the teat ends, should be well cleaned and completely dried, which will also help to reduce liner slips to a minimum.

To Wash or Not to Wash?

Over the years there has been much discussion as to whether the washing of all teats within a milking herd is necessary. In the summer months, when cattle are at pasture or in herds where the housing is particularly well managed and the teats are visibly clean, it has been argued that introducing water can have adverse effects on milk quality and possibly mastitis rates. However, one thing is certain and that is that, if you wash teats in preparation for milking, you must dry them. While washing is desirable, the mobilization of bacteria into a liquid, infectious soup will be deleterious to milk quality and will risk increasing mastitis rates if the teats are not dried. The teats are aligned vertically and so any water not removed by drying will run down the teat

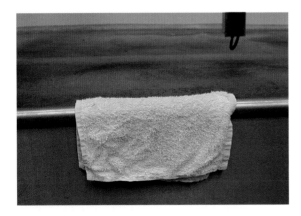

Flannel towel – single use, that is, one per cow; laundered and dried before reuse.

surface and off the end carrying bacteria with it directly into the milk intended for human consumption. The teat end will also effectively be bathed in this bacterial soup, which will significantly increase the potential for bacteria to enter the quarter through the streak canal, resulting in mastitis.

Despite the term 'udder washing' being used, it is more usual and effective to restrict the washing and drying procedure to just the teats. If the udder is very dirty, and particularly if the contamination is wet (for example, if a cow slips down and comes into the parlour with her udder bathed in faeces), then washing more than just the teats is acceptable and necessary. In this situation effective and thorough drying will be crucial because of the increased opportunity for larger volumes of contaminated water to drain into the teat cup liner as compared with when only the teat is washed. However, the time involved in drying the large area of washed udder is considerable and will severely reduce parlour cow throughputs. As a result, the benefits from managing housing hygienically so that cows enter the parlour clean will be self-evident.

Wet Teat Preparatory Procedures

Teat washing (with the above mentioned caveat of the requirement for drying) is very effective in controlling the bacterial count in milk. As with many disinfection scenarios, the physical washing process will remove a large percentage of bacteria from the teats. This can be summarized in the phrase 'the solution to pollution is dilution'. However, the addition of a disinfectant will help to further reduce pathogen numbers. Where chemicals are used they must be appropriate for the production of milk for human consumption and used at the correct concentration. If they are used in concentrations greater than those recommended by the manufacturer, they may cause damage to the teat skin and increase mastitis rates. Low-pressure sprayers are more convenient and generally more hygienic for washing udders than are buckets of water. Low-pressure sprayers that deliver a low volume of water are better than high-pressure sprayers that provide a high volume. Perhaps the most common method of teat preparation in milking parlours is to use a drop hose (delivering water containing disinfectant) and gloved hands to remove debris from teats, but avoiding wetting the udder beyond the area immediately surrounding the base of the teat. Enough water must be used to ensure good teat cleaning, making sure that the far side of the teat which cannot be easily seen is clean. However, the more water that is used will mean more to dry off the teats, as it will drain to this dependent point.

The use of a disinfectant wash solution in a bucket is not advisable because sponges and common cloths can easily transfer mastitis-causing pathogens to uninfected quarters and cows. A bucket of disinfectant wash solution does not kill all the bacteria present on a common udder cloth or sponge, particularly when the contamination has built up. It is possible to change the disinfectant wash solution regularly, but in reality this is rarely done frequently enough.

The 'ultimate', but extreme, wet preparation occurs where a sprinkler pen is used and mushroom caps over fire-extinguisher-type sprinklers soak the underside of the cows as they stand in the collecting yard, waiting to be milked. In theory, the time that the sprinkler is running can be adjusted to the degree of soiling of the udders. Sufficient 'drip drying' time prior to entering the parlour is critical, and once the cows are in the parlour it is essential that individual paper towels are used to finish the drying of udder and teats. This type of 'teat prep' tends to be used in larger herds in countries with a less inclement and warmer climate. The author has seen herds where this method was used with no further action being taken other than unit attachment once the cows have entered the parlour, and, not surprisingly, this resulted in high environmental mastitis rates.

Dry Teat Preparation/No Preparatory Procedures

To avoid potential problems from wet udders and teats and the extra time needed for drying, some milkers opt either to wipe teats with a dry hand (possibly gloved), dry towel or maybe use no preparation at all. While a badly performed job of washing and inadequate drying of teats and udders may be no better (and in some cases, worse) than no preparation, the best results are achieved from a first-rate job of cleaning and drying teats. Research in the USA has shown that even with cows whose teats look to be visibly clean there were from three to sixteen times more bacteria in the milk from 'no prep' cows, 'wet udder' cows, or

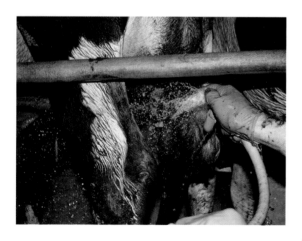

Dirty udder may need washing.

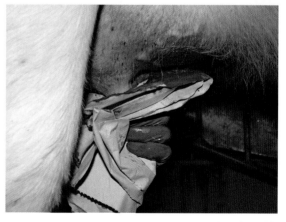

After washing, careful drying is essential.

'dry wipe' cows than from 'properly prepped' cows.

Ideal Teat Preparation

From this US research it was concluded that the best preparation was considered to be the use of either (1) a low-pressure drop hose and water with disinfectant used to clean the teats, only with some hand manipulation of the teats during washing (both vertical motion, say, three or four times to remove dirt and faeces from the teat, as well as horizontal motion, say, once or twice across the teat end to remove dirt and faeces from the teat end), followed by manual towel drying, or (2) a wet, individual, cow paper towel for cleaning the teats only, followed by manual towel drying. However, this work also indicates that pre-dipping teats plus manual drying with a paper or flannel towel and ensuring that the teat end is dried effectively can be as effective as a first-class job of washing teats with water (drop hose or wet towel) plus manual drying.

Other Options to Aid Teat Preparation

Removing hair from udders – clipping or flaming; long hair on udders should be removed regularly as dirt and faeces may adhere to the udder and make it more difficult to properly clean and dry teats. The hair can be removed with electric clippers, as can the tail hair, as a dirty tail, which is more often seen during winter housing, can soil the udder. Flaming or singeing udders (sometimes called 'low-heat clipping') can also be used to remove hairs. This is normally done with a butane or propane gas wand, which is a copper pipe approximately 1m in length attached to the gas cylinder by a flexible pipe and adjusted to allow sufficient air to the burner to create a cool orange flame to be used for singeing the hairs.

The removal of long hairs will not only help to keep dirt and faeces off udders and teat ends, reducing the need for extensive teat preparation and making milking time shorter, but it is likely to have added benefits in reducing bactoscan and mastitis rates. It would also be expected to help to contribute to reducing Johne's disease spread by reducing the chance of new-born calves becoming infected by sucking on contaminated teats.

Automation or Semi-automation of Teat Preparation

Automation of teat preparation is a requirement for AMS. AMS is covered in more detail on page 129. Semi-automatic teat preparation is also possible, using a hand-held washing unit containing motorized rotating brushes

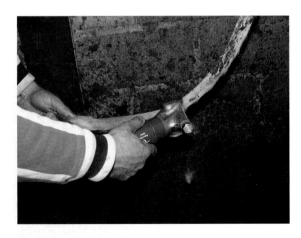

Electric clipper being used to remove hair from the tail during the winter housing period.

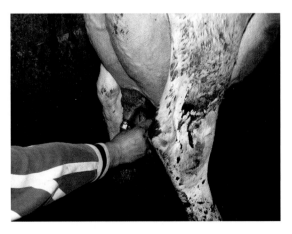

Clipper can also be used on udders to remove hair.

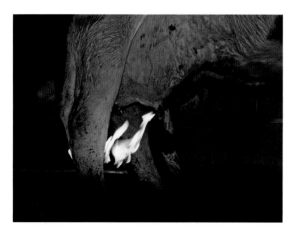

Udder singeing can be effective in removing hair from udders; it may need to be done two or three times during the winter housing period.

Electric brushes with plumbed sanitized water for teat preparation. They can be used without water flow after cleaning to dry the teats.

which wash, massage, disinfect and then dry the teats before milking. The massage provides some stimulation of the udder, possibly encouraging milk let-down. There are three brushes, with the upper two being counter-rotating which wash the external surface of the teat and the bottom of the udder, while the third

Arrangement of brushes within a hand-held, motorized brush unit for teat preparation.

brush washes the tip of the teat with sanitized water containing a rapidly acting disinfectant such as peracetic acid. Pressing the trigger under the handle of the washing unit starts the flow of sanitized water and the brushes to rotate. Each teat is washed for about 1sec by moving the washing unit vertically and rotating it clockwise and counterclockwise. When the trigger is released the water stops and the brushes then rotate faster and dry the teats which helps to avoid the contamination of the milk by not allowing dirty water to enter the liner once the units are attached. The sanitized water is piped to the brush head and so will be clean for each cow. The brushes have the potential to collect detritus and bacteria and so vigorous cleaning of the brush head periodically is a sensible precaution, as well as regular replacement of the brushes. The whole process of teat preparation is completed in 10 to 15sec per cow.

Pre-milking Teat Disinfection (PrMTD)

PrMTD can be delivered by either dipping the teats by the use of a teat-dip cup or by spraying by using a multipoint drop line spray system within the parlour. PrMTD is a relatively new development in milking time hygiene, unlike post-milking teat disinfection (PMTD), which

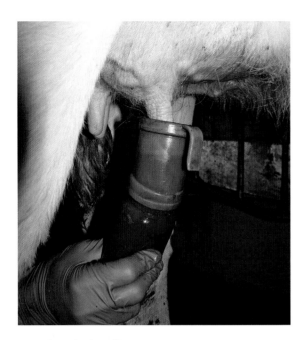

Teat disinfection dip cup.

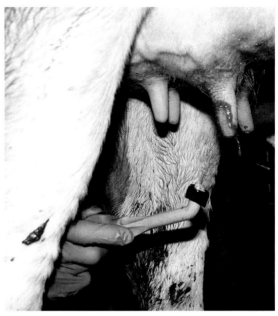

Teat disinfection spray line.

has been the cornerstone of milking routines for many years and is a key part of the NIRD five-point plan.

PMTD is primarily aimed at controlling contagious pathogens acquired during milking from infected milk from previously milked cows and has the secondary effect of improving teat skin condition, whereas PrMTD is primarily aimed at reducing the environmental pathogen load on the teat surface, which is generally acquired between milkings and also has a secondary effect of improving milk hygiene. Teat sanitizing by either PrMTD or PMTD will reduce, but not eliminate, mastitis-causing pathogens, resulting in a reduction of the chance of these pathogens penetrating the streak canal and causing new intrammmary infections. PMTD will have no effect on mastitis arising from contamination of teats acquired between milkings, so PrMTD has been applied in some herds to control environmental mastitis.

There are several advantages of PrMTD over disinfectant udder washing, most notably minimizing the amount of water used in teat preparation but still effectively reducing the

number of bacteria on the teat surface which may act as a source for mastitis cases. It is theorized that bacteria on the teat surface as the cow enters the parlour can act as a source for mastitis cases by being driven into the mammary gland with the milking machine contributing to the final common pathway. This insult can be by retrograde flow resulting in 'impacts' (milk impacting the teat end) during low initial or end flow rates when vacuum fluctuations are more common or via rapid movement of air into the clawpiece with liner slips. Cross-contamination can also occur when the teat ends are bathed in milk during 'flooding' of the clawpiece bowl, which tends to occur when there are very high milk flow rates and the parlour is temporarily unable to remove the milk from the clawpiece bowl.

If pre-dipping is going to be used, then manual drying of all four teats with an individual towel is essential not only to achieve reduced bacterial counts and sediment levels from dirt and faeces, but also to minimize the risk of potential disinfectant residues in milk. So, if manual drying is not used as part of the milking routine, then nor should pre-

107

dipping. Equally, if teats are contaminated with dirt or faeces such that pre-dipping with subsequent drying does not physically clean the teats, then they should be washed and dried before pre-dipping. The effectiveness of pre-dipping, like any disinfecting process, will be dependent upon the organic load (dirt and faeces) on the teat surface which will impede the ability to kill the bacteria present on the surface which have accumulated from exposure during the period between milkings. Work with both experimental bacterial challenge and natural exposure has shown that exposure to heavy environmental contamination, even shortly after milking, reduces the effectiveness of pre-dipping, whereas minimizing contamination by keeping cows clean for 1 to 2hr after milking will maximize the benefits from PrMTD.

Teat preparation including PrMTD is as follows:

- precleaning/washing of teats, as necessary
- forestripping (may be done before or after applying teat dip)
- dipping or spraying teats with a proven germicidal specific pre-dip product
- waiting the manufacturer's recommended contact time (usually 15 to 40sec)
- drying each teat, with particular attention to the teat end by using a single-service paper towel or laundered cloth towel to remove surplus dip (germicidal product), bacteria and organic material
- attachment of teat cups to the dry udder.

This is often shortened to: STRIP, DIP then DRY and APPLY.

Some people change the order of the above points and apply the pre-dip first, immediately forestripping and then waiting the recommended contact time before wiping and applying DIP, STRIP then DRY and APPLY. There might be additional benefits from this order as the massaging of the teat during forestripping might improve the effect of the pre-dip by encouraging the dip to penetrate into the teat skin and facilitate the removal of surface

bacteria, however, if, as is sometimes the case, pre-dipping is used without prior washing of teats and the dip is applied on top of faeces and dirt, the efficacy will be significantly reduced and there will also be an increased risk of disinfectant residues being present in the milk, and, further to this, it is unlikely to reduce the incidence of mastitis or lower the SCC and may well reduce milk quality; faeces and dirt must be removed to realise the full benefits of pre-dipping.

For proper coverage and effectiveness from dipping or spraying, all teats must be completely covered. Too often, the teats on the opposite side from the milker are inadequately dipped or sprayed. A minimum of 15 to 20sec for skin-contact time is needed for a pre-dip teat disinfectant to effectively kill bacteria. When environmental mastitis pathogens are at a high level on the teats, a skin-contact time of 30 to 40sec may be needed. In practice, pre-dipping takes 3 to 6sec per cow, manual drying 6 to 8sec and forestripping 4 to 7sec. Even if predipping with manual drying takes longer than simple rinsing with a water hose,

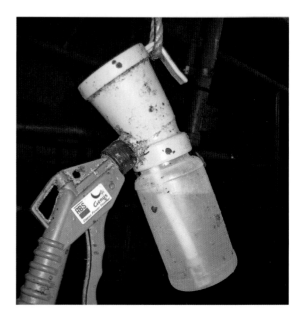

Foaming pre-milking teat disinfection delivery system.

the benefit of reducing environmental mastitis by up to 50 per cent may justify the practice, especially during wet, muddy weather, and if the cow's teats (and udder) are wet when entering the parlour. This extra manipulation can also result in enhanced milk letdown, resulting in shorter milking times.

The benefit PrMTD offers in reducing teat skin bacterial loads means that herds experiencing a problem with environmental mastitis should consider adopting this simple procedure. However, only products designated as pre-dips with proven efficacy should be used and always in strict accordance with the manufacturer's recommendations. More recently, foams and gels have been introduced for PrMTD which have the added advantage of further limiting the amount of water involved in teat preparation, making wiping with a single-service towel easier but still essential. However well it is performed, pre-dipping can never replace good teat preparation and is, in fact, only a part of good milking routine, and so at the end of milking, after the milking units have been removed, post-milking teat dipping should also be continued. When used in conjunction with all the other procedures in a good milking routine pre-dipping is an asset to a total mastitis control programme.

4. DRY TEATS

This is a critical part of the milking routine and has been covered in the teat preparation section. Suffice it to say here that drying after washing or the application of pre-milking teat disinfectant is crucial to producing high quality milk, avoiding chemical residues and helping to reduce mastitis rates. It is critical that the teat end is included in the drying process by wiping the paper or flannel towel over the teat and rolling it across the teat end.

Milk Let-down and Lag Times
The period between teat preparation and unit attachment is critical to ensure efficient, rapid and sustained milk flow. This period is commonly referred to as the 'lag time or 'prep lag

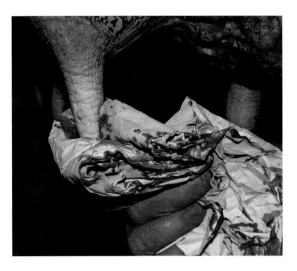

When wiping the teats, it is essential that the end is wiped.

time'. The prep lag time is the time between the beginning of teat preparation and the application of the milking machine and is aimed to coincide with the maximal oxytocin release. As a consequence, as the cisternal milk is removed by the milking machine it will be replaced by milk moving from the alveoli to the cistern, ensuring continuous flow.

If the prep lag is incorrect the initial flow of cisternal milk will not be followed by the movement of milk from the alveolar store to the udder cistern and milk flow may temporarily cease, followed by a reappearance of milk flow. This type of flow is described as bimodal and will be recognized as either a temporary slowing or, in extreme cases, a complete cessation of flow after the initial and immediate flow of cisternal milk. This will result in over-milking at the beginning of milking rather than as is more commonly seen at the end of each cow's milking. Over-milking is effectively the time the cow's teat is exposed to a high vacuum during low flow of milk and is probably more common at the beginning of milking (soon after unit attachment) in larger herds than at the end of milking, unlike in smaller herds and particularly those without ACRs.

It is thought that bimodal flow can result both from too long a prep lag time by the presence of cisternal milk inhibiting the oxy-tocin driven ejection of milk from the alveoli, or from too short a prep lag time in which case the cisternal milk is depleted before the alveolar milk has arrived. The amount of milk stored in the udder cistern accumulates between milking and so increases with the time between milkings. As a result, the amount of cisternal milk is relatively low during the first few hours after milking but then increases as the next milking approaches. Cisternal milk volumes vary with the cow's milk yield and consequently the stage of lactation. A late lactation cow may hold as little as 1 to 2ltr of cisternal milk, while a fresh calved cow may yield around 3 to 4ltr of cisternal milk.

It is clear that the prep lag time is an extremely important factor in optimizing milking efficiency and, despite the fact that the optimal prep lag time will vary with cow yield and so will depend on the stage of lactation, it is generally accepted that between 60 and 90sec is optimal across all stages of lactation.

In a well sorted milking routine where milk let-down and flow are optimized as are both the amount of preparation and the prep lag time, unit-on time and low flow/high vacuum periods can be reduced. It is said in the USA that for a typical dairy cow, an investment of 20sec in teat preparation will reduce the average unit-on time by 90sec. Although difficult to demonstrate experimentally, reduced unit-on time should benefit both cow (teats exposed to fewer pulsation phases, resulting in less teat end damage, such as hyperkeratosis) and operator (milking will take less time).

5. UNIT ATTACHMENT

Proper unit attachment is extremely important. Once the cow has been prepared, the milking units should be attached carefully and consistently, minimizing stress to the cows and preventing excessive air from entering the milking system. Some air entering the plant at unit attachment is unavoidable but it should be kept to a minimum. The amount of air entering can easily be gauged because it is

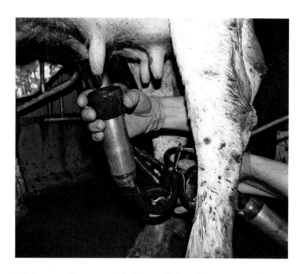

Unit attachment – kinking of the short milk tube ensures that little air is admitted.

clearly audible. When each teat cup is attached the short milk tube should be kinked over on the bevel on the clawpiece (*see* photo above) prior to attachment to avoid air rushing into the plant rather than just 'folding' it up, which will allow air to rush in and cause vacuum fluctuations. As individual teat cups are attached the teat cup is raised up toward the teat and the short milk tube is straightened out to minimize air admission to the system.

6. Unit Adjustment

Once the units have been attached the milker should check and make adjustments if necessary before moving on to the next cow. Ideally, the claw should be as horizontal as possible, with the outlet of the claw perhaps pointing in a slightly downward direction to facilitate milk flow into the long milk tube and away from the cow. Good unit adjustment will minimize liner slips, especially toward the end of milking and contribute to overall milking efficiency. Different parlour configurations have different milking unit set-ups such that the long milk tube and long pulsation tubes may be 'between the legs' or 'in front of the legs', which creates different issues in stabilizing and aligning the clawpieces. Some parlours have special clips or support arms which hold the long milk tube to help to maintain ideal clawpiece alignment, with some milkers improvising and making bespoke clips with coathanger wire.

Cows with large, pendulous udders can be difficult to milk as the short milk tubes are not long enough to reach from clawpiece to teat effectively. This can cause difficulty in correct clawpiece alignment and liner slips can also occur as the liners cannot be placed correctly on the teats. Extensions to the short milk tube can help to correct this by allowing the liners to reach all four teats.

Milking Sequence

The time taken to milk a herd (measured as cows milked per hour) completely will be influenced most by the number of operators milking and the number of milking units in the parlour. In abreast or tandem parlours, where a one-in-one-out principle applies, the time to milk an individual cow can be adjusted without impacting the time to milk other cows. However, reducing the total time to milk the whole herd is difficult. Equally, any extra time added to the routine, such as PrMTD or cluster disinfection, will be multiplied by the number of cows milked as no time can be 'shared'. In

herringbone or rotary parlours the cows milked per hour can also be influenced by the way the milking procedures (strip, dip, dry and apply) are applied, particularly when there is more than one operator. Much has been written on the way milking procedures are applied to groups of cows in larger parlours in order to increase parlour throughputs. Effectively, there are two main options where either all the cows in the parlour have the milking procedures applied one after another as a batch or they can be subdivided into groups within the parlour and the procedures applied one after another within that group. The influence of different strategies on parlour throughput in terms of cows milked per hour depends on the number of milkers and becomes more significant the larger the parlour. In more modern, larger, high throughput parlours one operator cannot keep up with milking and so multiple operators are becoming more common. There are four main ways to approach the application of milking procedures within a parlour routine (*see* table overleaf).

The type of routine needs to be matched to the number of cows to be milked, the teat preparation time, the type of parlour (abreast, tandem, herringbone or rotary), the number of

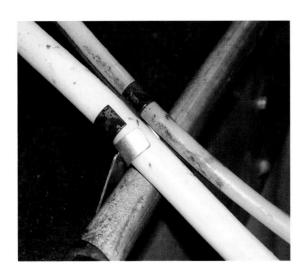

Long milk tube clip to aid good cluster alignment.

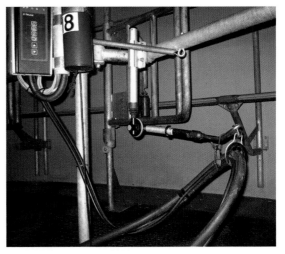

Long milk tube support arm to aid good cluster alignment.

111

milkers available and the number of standings and units in the parlour (swing-over parlours versus equivalent doubled-up parlours). The aim is to optimize the lag time to give good milk let-down such that milking out of cisternal milk is followed by alveolar milk without a bimodal pattern, thus avoiding over-milking and minimizing teat-end eversion and assuming ACRs are correctly set for unit detachment.

Milking Order

Cows are creatures of habit and will often prefer one side of a herringbone parlour to the other. The order in which cows enter the parlour to be milked is more complex and is affected by many factors including social status, milk yields and parity number. Parity number, a proxy measure of (milking) age, is linked to social status to a certain extent. Cattle have a hierarchical social structure within a group such as a milking herd and respect an order for feeding which is often similar to the order for entering the milking parlour. Manipulating the milking order can be a useful technique to try to protect uninfected cattle from acquiring infection from infected cattle via fomite spread within the parlour. One must remember that, however good a milking routine is, there is always a chance of infection spread to cows milked after an infected cow within a herd during milking. The impact of changing the milking order on mastitis spread within a herd will depend on how many infected cows exist in the herd. This will also determine the impact on the milker's time to achieve it. In its simplest form it might involve milking two or three known infected cows last to running a separate 'dirty' group.

Although not popular in the modern dairy, herd segregating the 'clean', uninfected cows and milking them first as a group before the high SCC infected cows can be a useful way of reducing the spread of infection within the herd. There are some limitations in the several methods of allocating cows as 'clean' or 'dirty', including accuracy, cost and speed of results. SCC from a composite milk sample

Milking sequence routines

Type of routine	Method
Batch	Generally only one operator All cows have each component procedure of the milking routine performed one cow after another before returning to the first cow and the next procedure is started. This can lead to extended lag times and bimodal milk flow in long herringbone parlours
Sequential	Sequential milking routine occurs when one milker performs a component procedure of the milking routine one cow after another but another milker follows (before the first milker has finished) applying the next milking procedure such that milking units are attached, the cows milked, the units detached and then the cows released
Territorial	Territorial routine differs in that one milker performs all procedures on all cows within one territory for say 6 to 8 cows at a time. This can apply to one milker working their way up one side of a parlour in territorial aliquots in an attempt to avoid extended lag times or to multiple milkers who deal only with the cows in their own territory
Group	Group milking routine is seen in very large parlours and is similar to a territorial routine but each milker will attend multiple territories and perform all the procedures within these territories

(commingled milk from all four quarters) is the most accessible to milkers but is generally available only monthly from routine milk recording data. CMT can be used at a quarter level and more frequently if desired but is time-consuming, particularly if several cows need checking. The author has found that, even with the limitations of composite SCC and infrequent measurement, significant improvement in mastitis rates and BMSCC can be achieved. When managing these groups a pragmatic approach is needed when allocating cows of uncertain status to either the clean or the dirty group. Although the concept has always been that of running a dirty group by using a SCC threshold of say 300 to 400,000 cells/ml, it may be best to think of running a clean group by using a SCC threshold of say 150 or even 100,000 cells/ml. In that way the increased confidence that cows within this clean group are uninfected will help to ensure that infected cows are not allocated to the clean group, allowing them to spread their infection within the clean group. With this approach there is, of course, a chance that a few clean cows may be allocated to the dirty group and condemned to running the gauntlet of acquiring infection from dirty cows. However, if the dirty group approach is taken and only cows that can confidently be identified as dirty are included in the dirty group, then some infected cows inevitably will be allocated to the clean group resulting in an unwanted spread of infection to uninfected cows. The use of the segregation of clean and dirty cows is by no means an exact science and, even with the limitations of correct identification and allocation to the right group, the significant reduction in the chance of milking clean cows after dirty cows will help to reduce new infection rates.

Milking Frequency

Cows are generally milked twice a day in the modern dairy herd, although some high-yielding herds may be milked three times a day. There are increased costs in feed and labour involved with three times a day milking and the increased profit will depend on the milk price and the magnitude of the increased yields and so may not always be justified. When milk quotas were a significant part of UK milk production some herds would use three times a day milking to increase yields to ensure that the farm, and to some extent the United Kingdom, achieved their quota. It must be remembered that part of the increased milk yield will be driven by better feeding and management and to a certain extent increased appetites and not just the reduced udder pressure and the removal of the negative feedback protein. In some larger, high-yielding herds where cattle are grouped by yield, three times a day milking is used only in the early lactation high-yielding group, where the benefits of reduced mastitis rates are likely to be more significant. The response to three times a day milking will be variable, but generally mastitis rates will be lower in herds milked three times daily and yields will increase by between 10 and 20 per cent. The proportional increase in yield will, however, be greatest in late lactation cows if three times a day milking is maintained throughout a lactation. The reduction in mastitis can be reflected in lower clinical mastitis rates as well as reduced SCC. Conversely, if cows are milked once a day yields will fall by 40 to 50 per cent and the SCC will generally rise, although if one milking is omitted in a week (in some countries a Sunday milking for social or religious reasons) this fall will be in the region of 5 to 10 per cent.

The increase in milk yield has both immediate and longer-term mechanisms. There is an immediate effect within days or even hours through the removal of back pressure and chemical feedback inhibitor increasing milk secretion. In the longer term, increased prolactin levels over days to weeks are associated with a stimulation of cell differentiation, which increases actual milk secretion, which, over weeks to months, results in the stimulation of cell proliferation which further increases milk secretion.

Milking Interval

The milking interval is generally determined by social factors and consequently a 10hr and a 14hr interval (often termed 10–14 milking schedule) is more common than a 12–12 schedule. Intervals of longer than 14hr do cause an overall reduction in milk production as back-pressure starts to affect milk secretion. A 10–14 interval allows the milker to finish the evening milking at a reasonable time without having to get up too early in the morning. There are few data to show that overall milk yield is significantly affected by a more even 12–12 interval. The longer interval of, say 14hr between an evening and morning interval will, of course, mean that the yield at the morning milking will be greater than the shorter inter-milking interval at the evening milking. Unlike yield, there is good evidence that BMSCC varies with different milking intervals. Longer intervals tend to have lower SCCs partly due to back pressure reducing cell diapedesis and partly due to the increased absolute yield, with a longer inter-milking interval resulting in greater dilution of somatic cells present and so morning milkings tend to have lower SCCs than evening milkings. This may also be a factor in a complex and not fully understood mechanism whereby AMS systems tend to have slightly higher SCCs as the milking interval, although variable, will average out shorter than conventional twice daily milking as there are often around 2.5 milkings per cow per day.

7. UNIT REMOVAL

After the milking for each cow is completed the unit can be removed. This can be done either manually or automatically.

Manual Unit Removal

With manual unit removal the milk flow for each cow being milked needs to be closely monitored and, when the milker considers the cow has finished milking the vacuum to that unit must be shut off first before the unit can be removed. Clips were used in older parlours without ACRs, however, some milkers shut off the vacuum by kinking the long milk tube, particularly in lower yield 'New Zealand-style' batch calving herds milked in large, low

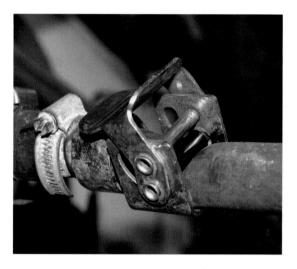

Manual clip use in parlours without ACRs to shut off the vacuum before the unit removal.

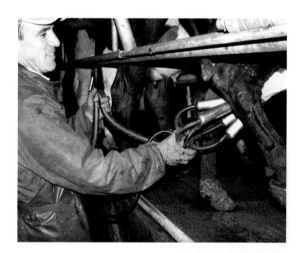

Some milkers, particularly in low vacuum parlours, kink the long milk tube before removing the unit.

vacuum parlours. Generally though, manual systems rely on good milker observation and so flow rates at unit removal will tend to vary, which increases the chance of either over- or under-milking.

Automatic Unit Removal: Automatic Cluster Removal System (ACR)

With automatic removal the vacuum is shut off and the unit removed by an ACR system at a given flow rate, often termed the switch point since this is when the ACR activates; however, there is also a standardized delay before unit removal. In some but not all parlours both the switch point and the delay can be adjusted, giving different degrees of milking out and resulting in different unit-on time and milk left in the udder (strip yields). A cow is commonly considered sufficiently milked when the flow rate drops below 200ml/min; however, the actual point of unit removal will vary depending on the delay setting for the ACR. The accuracy of the delay setting will differ with the make and actual settings of the ACR, resulting in delay times probably being the most inconsistent factor among types of ACR. So although manufacturers have settings for parlour installations, switch points and delay times are probably best evaluated once the parlour is being used on farm.

Over- and Under-milking: ACR Settings and Strip Yields

Removal of all the milk from the udder is not desirable, particularly as the time and effort required to milk out the last few millilitres will extend unit-on time, exposing the teats to the prolonged effects of vacuum and pulsation, reducing parlour throughput and extending the time milkers spend milking their herd. Conversely, if units are removed prematurely this will leave more milk in the udder than is desirable and, in extreme cases, this can reduce milk yields. The amount of milk remaining in the udder at the end of milking in any parlour may be monitored by hand stripping a few cows immediately after milking for a maximum of 1min (15sec per quarter). This volume of milk is called the 'strip yield' and will be influenced by switch points and delay settings of ACRs. The set-up of a parlour in terms of milking out and ACR settings can be checked and parlours can be monitored by checking strip yields from a few cows at different stages of lactation. Strip yields of between 150 and 250ml evenly distributed between the quarters indicate that the cows are being well milked out, although some work shows that strip yields as low as 100ml per cow are acceptable in some high-yielding cows.

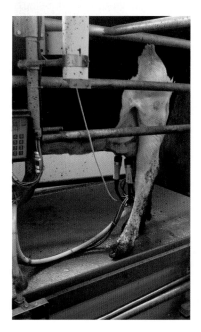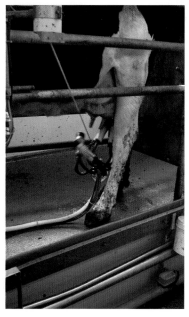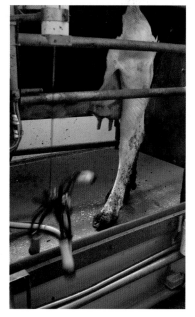

ACR sequence showing cluster removal.

115

However, the proportion of cows with significantly more than 250ml of strip yield should not be above 10 per cent or under-milking is an issue which may well be impacting cow yields. Over-milking however can be detected by looking for a few key indicators as well as finding low strip yields. Such signs of over-milking might include teat discoloration and ringing at the base of the teat after unit detachment, restless or kicking cows, particularly towards the end of each cow's milking when flow rates are low, with the possibility of the long milk tubes or clawpieces containing no milk. Remember that some of these behavioural signs such as restlessness and kicking at the unit can be seen at the beginning of milking where over-milking can occur with poor unit-on lag times resulting in bimodal milk flow (*see* milk let-down and lag times above under '4. Dry Teats'). The consequences of longer-term over-milking occur because the teats are repeatedly milked while becoming empty of milk towards the end of each cow's milking and this can result in hyperkeratosis or teat-end eversions. If over-milking is suspected it may be worth increasing the ACR threshold values and/or decreasing the delay time in small steps until the signs disappear. Several studies, including work done in Denmark, have shown that if the switch point is increased from a very commonly used setting of 200ml/min flow rate to 400ml/min and the delay time decreased from 12 to 7sec, the machine-on time is reduced from 7.8 to 6.4min and the milk production increased slightly from 39 to 40kg per cow per day. Consequently, trends within the dairy industry are for ACRs to be set for higher flow rates at unit take-off, with shorter delays from the switch point ('wet milking') resulting in shorter unit-on time and thus increasing parlour throughput without impacting milk yields.

Machine Stripping

Machine stripping is not to be recommended but is facilitated when downward pressure is applied to the cluster bowl towards the end of milking, either in the form of weights (historically old ploughshares) or by placing a hand on the bowl, and is often accompanied by hand massaging to encourage further milkout. This practice is likely to result in both over-milking, with the associated increased risk of hyperkeratosis as well as increasing the risk of liner slips, which, in turn, will increase the likelihood of new intramammary infections.

Dealing with Cows with Mastitis

If cows are identified as having mastitis (*see* Chapter 3) their milk is diverted from the bulk supply by the use of a dump line, dump bucket or via a tap at the bottom of the recorder jar to ensure it is not submitted for human consumption. The cow identity, quarter involved, date, batch number and treatment used should all be recorded. Often the cow is identified with a stock spray marker or the use of coloured tail tape. Once the milking unit is removed

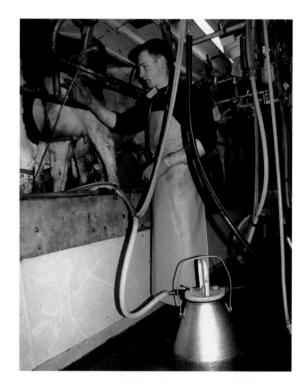

Dump bucket used for milking cows (such as mastitis cows) producing milk not intended to go into the bulk tank.

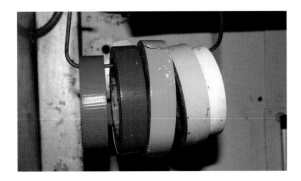

Tail tape is often used to identify treated cows to remind the milker that their milk needs to be discarded.

any cows identified as suffering from a case of mastitis can receive the appropriate treatment (*see* Chapter 7).

8. POST-MILKING TEAT DISINFECTION

Reducing Infection Spread

Disinfection of teat skin after milking (post-milking disinfection) will reduce the chance of any bacteria transferred to the teats via contaminated milking equipment from previous cows milked earlier from entering the udder and setting up an infection. This infection pressure can also be reduced by removing infected quarters within the herd by treating those infected quarters during lactation or at drying off in cattle, where the chance of success is believed to be good, or by drying off infected quarters or culling problem cows, where it is not. As the milking machine itself acts as a fomite and facilitates infection spread from an infected cow to other cows subsequently milked through this same cluster unit, disinfection of the cluster and, more specifically, the liners, can also be useful in reducing this chance of spread. The ability of any bacteria to behave in a contagious manner is not necessarily innate, but merely the fact that the more persistent an infection within the udder or on the teat skin the greater chance of fomite spread from one cow to another (or,

in fact, from one quarter to another). As a consequence, the contagious spread of any bacteria, even say *E. coli*, might be seen where a cow is milked through the same cluster subsequent to a clinical case of mastitis shedding huge numbers of bacteria into the milk. Often in this situation a contagious pathogen such as *Staphylococcus aureus* can be detected within the liner after milking from six to eight cows following a cow known to be infected.

Post-milking Teat Disinfection

The aim of post-milking teat disinfection (PMTD) is both to disinfect the teats after the cow has been milked, killing bacteria acquired from the milking parlour and originating from infected quarters in previous cows milked earlier, as well as to improve teat condition. The type of chemical, concentration and level of emollient or humectant (teat conditioners) such as lanolin or glycerine used will vary from product to product. There will, however, be a compromise in the formulation, as increasing the teat conditioners will, in general, reduce the killing ability of the disinfectant, whereas increasing the concentration of disinfectant will tend to adversely affect the teat skin condition. Similarly, good, well moisturized teat skin will be able to resist colonization by bacteria more readily, helping to reduce mastitis rates. So, depending on the prevalence of contagious pathogens within a herd (indirectly indicated by BMSCC) and the current teat skin condition, the importance of high levels of either teat conditioner or disinfectant may be the priority. Barrier dips are a more recent development and are aimed to give better control over environmental bacterial challenge between milkings by sealing the teat end. The difficulty is finding a product that will persist (ideally, between milkings) but be easily removed by normal teat preparation. Products based on barrier technology have often produced a 'plastic skin' which can flake off, plug milk filters and cause cleaning problems. More recently, products have been formulated to give a rapid initial kill and produce a moist, waxy film that covers the teat orifice and remains soft and flexible while still protecting against bacterial growth. Some products claim that the activity is maintained even after the dip has dried to the waxy state, particularly when the product is rehydrated when cows lie in moist bedding, mud and faeces or when they encounter rain and the germicidal activity is reactivated.

In general, post-milking teat disinfection most commonly takes the form of either manual spraying or dipping of the teat skin, with some more recent approaches attempting to automate the application of the disinfectant to the skin. In manual systems disinfectants are applied to the teat surface as soon as possible after the milking cluster is removed, and this is critical to minimize the potential for bacteria transferred on to the teat surface from contaminated milking equipment to gain access to the mammary gland via the streak canal. Some dip cup systems have been developed to reduce the contamination of the disinfectant from detritus on the teat surface and reduce disinfectant wastage by spillage. These teat dip cups have two chambers with a reservoir below and the functional dip cup on top. The reservoir is squeezed to fill the cup and, after the teats have been dipped, the disinfectant returns by negative pressure to the reservoir. These two-chambered systems have the added advantage of being unable to be spilled if the teat cup is knocked over in the parlour. Teat spraying is generally a 'plumbed in' system where multiple 'drop lines' are positioned in the parlour such that all cows can be reached. They produce a relatively fine spray of disinfectant which, when applied correctly, covers the teat surface. In non-bespoke systems some people have adapted garden or greenhouse sprays which are hand-held and carried around the parlour from cow to cow. In general, the accepted wisdom is that dipping is more effective than spraying and this will be in part due to the fact that spraying is more prone to ineffective application, resulting in poor teat surface coverage. If done correctly, spraying will use more teat dip at 15ml per cow, compared with 10ml for dipping.

Automation of PMTD

Automation can take the form of an external system directing the disinfectant by a spray to the teat surface or, more recently, developments have seen the delivery of disinfectant to the teat surface from within the teat liner.

Automatic PMTD Outside the Parlour

Initial developments to automate the delivery of disinfectant to the teat surface were by floor-mounted spray nozzles to direct the disinfectant on to the teat surface. These were generally sited outside the parlour on a low, horizontal bar, generally a stainless steel tube aligned longitudinally and centrally in the exit passageway with a spray nozzle pointing upwards. There are several disadvantages to these systems and as a result they did not become popular. The inevitable delay between cluster removal and the application of the disinfectant, because they are generally sited a little way down the exit passageway from the parlour to avoid disturbance to the cow flow,

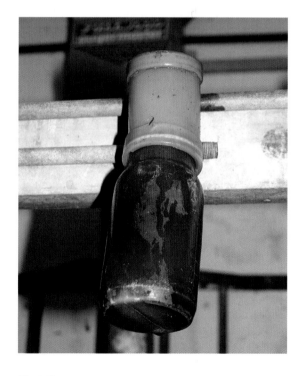

Teat dip cup.

118

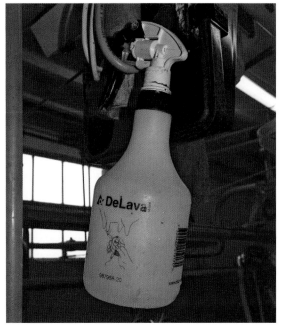

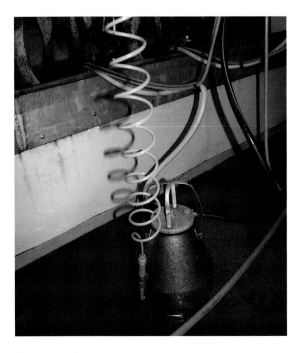

Teat spray line.

Hand-held spray.

is not ideal. Cows have to pass the bar as they travel down the passageway and, although they become accustomed to it, there can be a degree of reticence followed by rushing, which can affect the accuracy of spray delivery, which is triggered by a magic eye detecting the cow as she moves down the passageway. As a result, disinfectant delivery is often

not consistent and it is not uncommon for coverage of the teat surface to be incomplete or for the teats to be missed altogether, let alone covering the all-important teat end.

Automatic PMTD Within the Parlour
More recent developments to automate PMTD (other than the well developed AMS systems)

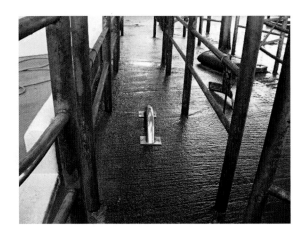

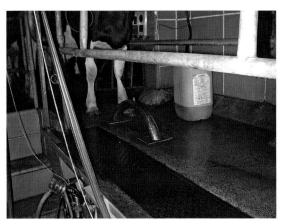

Automatic post-milking teat spray.

Automatic spray adapted for pre-milking spraying.

have been by encompassing the system within the milking machine itself.

Automatic Disinfection and Flushing (ADF)

One such system is Automatic Disinfection and Flushing (ADF), made by Research Development and Innovations Ltd (RDI). With ADF, the disinfectant and subsequent flush is applied through a small nozzle near the mouthpiece of a specially designed liner, via an extra pipe which runs inside a bespoke liner shell and is connected to the clawpiece. The disinfectant and flush water or sanitized water is delivered to the clawpiece by an extra pipe alongside the long milk and pulsation tubes. Once the milk flow has fallen below a configurable threshold, the vacuum is switched off by the ACR system and the teats receive a squirt of teat dip before the cluster is removed. As the ACR removes the cluster, the teats are effectively wiped with teat dip and, despite the low volume of dip, usually 6 to 8ml, gravity ought to ensure that some dip should reach the critical area of the teat end. The disinfectant not only disinfects the teat immediately prior to cluster removal but also floods the surface of the liners with disinfectant, albeit for a short contact time before flushing the system with water or, with more recent installations, a sanitized solution, most commonly peracetic acid. The flushing action is essential to ensure that there are no residues of disinfectant within the cluster, which would, if present, contaminate the milk from the next cow to be milked. The flushing and compressed air blast is repeated six times, with the first flush showing significant milk and dip residues being flushed out (*see* automatic cluster disinfection and flushing later in this chapter).

Clearly, avoiding disinfectant residues in milk intended for human consumption is very important, and, until the technology had been developed to achieve both disinfection and flushing, the industry generally had to rely on manual systems. The automation of the teat disinfection with ADF has a number of potential benefits. It removes the human

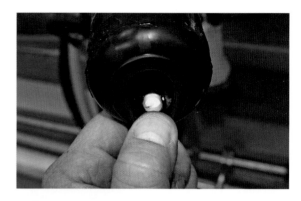

ADF release valve.

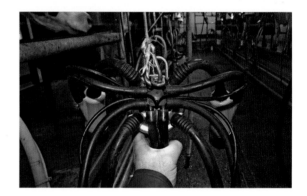

ADF clawpiece.

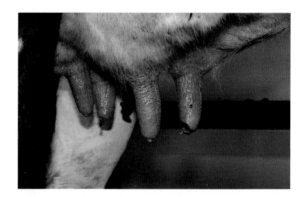

ADF teats dipped.

intervention, thus ensuring that it is performed to a given standard in terms of timing after each cow is milked, the volume of disinfectant used and teat coverage. It also releases the milker from the job of PMTD, allowing for greater attention to other parts of the milking routine,

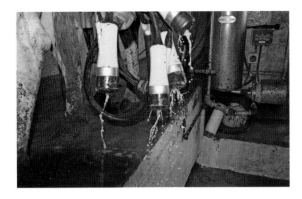

ADF first flush; note the teat dip chemical residue in the flush.

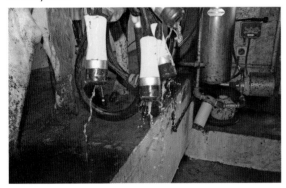

ADF subsequent flush.

and may in many parlours increase the parlour throughput in terms of cows milked per hour. It might be worth noting that, unlike many conventional clawpieces, the ACR cord is attached to the top of the ADF clawpiece rather than the bottom, so that the unit hangs the right way up for unit attachment, precluding the need to rotate the unit when it is attached. Automated systems require accurate setting up otherwise they consistently underperform. The timing of vacuum shut off, delivery of teat dip and removal of cluster are critical to ensure good teat coverage, avoidance of teat-end trauma on cluster removal and effective flushing of the cluster ready for the next cow. This is controlled by the ADF control box.

In some ways there may be a compromise in the choice of teat dip, particularly in water flush installations where there is a degree of reliance on cluster disinfection from the teat dip. Where the cluster disinfection is being more effectively delivered by a peracetic acid flush, the choice of teat dip can be aimed more at a longer duration of activity with more teat conditioning effects. This will be somewhat similar to the arguments against using a combined pre- and post-milking disinfectant. The requirements of a disinfectant for use in liner disinfection are broadly similar to those for a

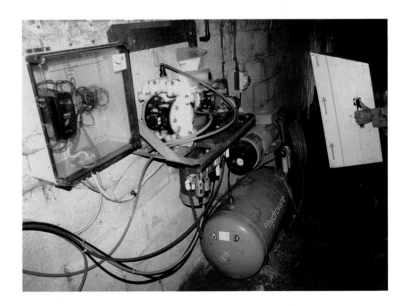

ADF control box.

pre-dip. A rapid kill is required since contact time will be short, particularly with liner disinfection as the chemical is flushed out almost immediately to allow the next cow to be milked. The compromise between speed and duration of activity is avoidable when choosing teat dips by using different products with a different speed of onset and duration of activity for pre- and post-milking disinfection.

However, with ADF, where a plain water flush is being used, one product is to a certain extent effectively doing two jobs which cannot be separated. The products for ADF are usually selected to ensure a useful post-dip action and any extra activity on the liners during the periods between application and flushing is effectively a bonus; however, it must be remembered that this is clearly better than doing nothing to disinfect clusters between cows, which is, in effect, what most parlours do. This is further discussed under post-milking cluster (liner) disinfection. Most ADF installations now have a disinfected water flush (most commonly peracetic acid) to improve the rapid disinfection of liners between cows. This has the advantage of separating the delivery to the teat surface via the special liner of a disinfectant after each cow is milked, where a persistent teat-conditioning product can be used, from the delivery of a rapid kill effect of, say, peracetic acid to disinfect the liners between each cow that is milked. This automated approach, particularly to the post-milking teat disinfection, assumes even more importance in an industry where the time pressures in the parlour are mounting as herd sizes increase and more cows are being milked per hour per operator. Much of the dairy industry around the world is seeing this increase in herd size and it is often coupled with low cost and relatively unskilled labour, which makes the quality control of certain tasks, such as teat disinfection and cluster removal by automation, even more attractive. However, it must be borne in mind that, if the equipment is not adequately maintained, it can equally become consistently substandard. This would result in the potential

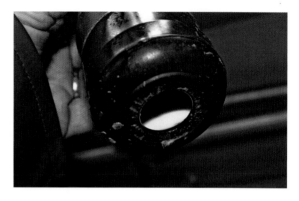

Milk residue in liner mouth piece immediately after a cow has been milked.

for the clusters to be removed at an inappropriate milk flow in the case of ACRs or the disinfection of the cow's teats particularly, and, to some extent, the liners to be ineffective in the case of ADF, both of which could result in increased mastitis rates. Automated systems in any area of life promise to be labour-saving, provided that they are set up correctly; if not, you can guarantee that they will inexorably and consistently do the job badly.

After an infected cow has been milked there will be residues of infected milk left within the milking apparatus and, when this comes into contact with the next cow to be milked, either by direct contact or indirectly by the movement of infected milk, there is a chance that infection will be transmitted to one of the quarters of up to the next six to eight cows. This type of indirect spread from cow to cow is via an object and is called fomite spread. The milker's hands or, indeed, a multi-use udder cloth, if one were inadvisably used, could equally spread mastitis bacteria from cow to cow.

Post-milking Cluster (Liner) Disinfection/Flushing

In general, a good hygienic milking routine will help to reduce the spread of infection from cow to cow. Historically, the risk of the spread of infection, by either the milker's hands or via wiping or drying teats with multi-use cloths or towels, has been reduced by wearing gloves and by ensuring that single-use cloths or towels are used. Additionally, the disinfection of liners between cows will help to reduce fomite spread of mastitis pathogens from cow to cow via the milking machine and is, perhaps, one area not covered well by the five-point plan. The five-point plan tended to concentrate on the disinfection of the teat surface immediately after milking (PMTD) to kill any bacteria transferred from the milking equipment to the teat surface during milking before they have a chance to gain entry to the quarter via the streak canal and set up an infection.

Although PMTD is still a critical and essential control point in any mastitis control programme and the wearing of gloves and single-use cloths or towels are important, the use of cluster disinfection, which has gained in popularity in recent years, is another way of trying to reduce fomite spread of infection from one cow to others subsequently milked through the same unit. This generally involves repeated application of disinfectant to the insides of the liners, effectively flushing the units clean and sanitizing them and will tend to augment the general principles of a good milking routine, which are themselves aimed at reducing the chance of spread of infection from cow to cow during the normal milking process. Cluster disinfection, while often manually applied, is becoming increasingly installed in both new and existing milking parlours as automated systems. When automatic flushing systems are observed, it is surprising how much residual milk is still present from the previous cow and is flushed from each unit. Up to 2 to 3ml of milk may be left in each liner and will act as a significant source of bacteria to infect the next cow to be milked.

You can see it if you look at the mouthpiece of a liner after a cow has been milked, provided that the liner is pointing down to allow the milk to accumulate at the mouthpiece. After an infected cow has been milked, this residue of infected milk left within the milking apparatus will come into contact with the next cows to be milked, either by direct contact or indirectly by the movement of infected milk over the liner surface, and there

is a chance that infection will be transmitted to one of the quarters of up to the next six to eight cows milked through that unit. Clearly, it is immaterial how efficient teat preparation and disinfection are before milking if teats are then inserted into liners bathed in milk containing potential mastitis-causing bacteria. This becomes even more critical in situations where milk let-down is delayed by poor cow stimulation from inadequate teat preparation and inappropriate unit-on lag times, giving rise to vacuum fluctuations which encourage retrograde milk flow, tending to drive bacterial contamination through the streak canal and increasing the chance of new intramammary infections. The most common disinfectant used is the hydrogen peroxide-based product peracetic acid at a very weak dilution of between 500:1 (0.2 per cent), using 50ml of peracetic acid in a 25ltr drum of water, up to a dilution of 200:1 (0.5 per cent), using 125ml

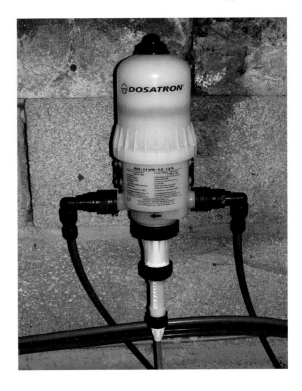

Dosing pump to deliver a known concentration of sanitizing solution (most often peracetic acid).

in a 25ltr drum. Often farms use something in between, say, 80ml in a 25ltr drum, or just over 0.3 per cent. There are serious considerations of milk residues when performing either pre-milking teat dipping/spraying or cluster disinfection, and it is best to take advice on which products and what concentrations to use. Special dosing pumps are increasingly being fitted to milking parlours to deliver a known concentration of sanitizing solution for either manual application or the automated systems described in this chapter. If excessive concentrations of flush are used it is possible that bulk milk could fail an inhibitory substance test (often incorrectly termed an antibiotic test), *see* Appendix I. What is clear, however, is that conventional post-milking teat disinfectants are ineffective for either pre-milking disinfection or for cluster disinfecting and will almost certainly produce unacceptable milk residues if used.

Manual Cluster Disinfection

Manual methods for cluster disinfection include dipping the liners in disinfectant, spraying a disinfectant inside each individual liner and, on occasions, backflushing with either water or sanitized water, although the latter is more commonly used for the control of bacterial spread after an individual mastitis case or known very high SCC cow is milked rather than a protocol used after all cows. Manual (as opposed to automatic) backflushing is only really possible in recorder jar milking parlours where the sanitizing solution can be captured in the recorder jar, drained and then flushed with water. The simple dipping of clusters in a bucket has several disadvantages, including the fact that the disinfectant is unlikely to penetrate up to the base of the liner due to air pressure build up, much as one would see if a jam jar were inverted and dipped in a bucket of water. There is an air bleed in the clawpiece which one might expect would facilitate the penetration of disinfectant; however, it is very small and the air released is insignificant in the time available to improve the movement of disinfectant up the liners.

There are ways of overcoming this restricted air expulsion limiting penetration of sanitizing solution by either dipping one or two liners at a time by 'jug dipping' or 'alternate dipping', which allows air to be rapidly expelled through the liners not being dipped.

Jug Dipping (see photos opposite)
One shell at a time is dipped in a somewhat similar fashion to teat dipping in a jug of sanitizing solution (collected from an already made up bucket or 'swing bin' of solution), while the cluster is suspended by the ACR cord. This also has the advantage that the cluster is at a workable height and precludes the need to drop the cluster to the floor to reach a bucket, which, if the ACR cord is too short, may require removal of the cord from the cluster for each cow, which is clearly time-consuming.

Alternate Dipping (see photos overleaf)
An alternative that the author finds useful, and can be quicker provided that the cluster can be dropped to reach a bucket without detaching the ACR cord, is to dip two liners inside a bucket while allowing two to remain outside the bucket, and then repeating the process by allowing the dipped liners to stay outside the bucket while the two undipped ones are dipped in the bucket. Care must be taken to select a bucket that ensures that the mouthpiece of the liners do not touch the ground while outside the bucket, although a standard 'yellow' bucket is generally sufficiently tall to avoid this.

With any dipping method, although a significant amount of potentially contaminated milk will gravitate to the mouthpiece and be flushed out, the base of the liner adjacent to the small milk tube will be at the top and difficult to reach since the cluster is upside down when it is dipped in the disinfectant and any bacterial contamination left there will be close to where the teat end of the next cow would lie during milking. A further problem with cluster dipping is that the bucket is prone to contamination with both the milk

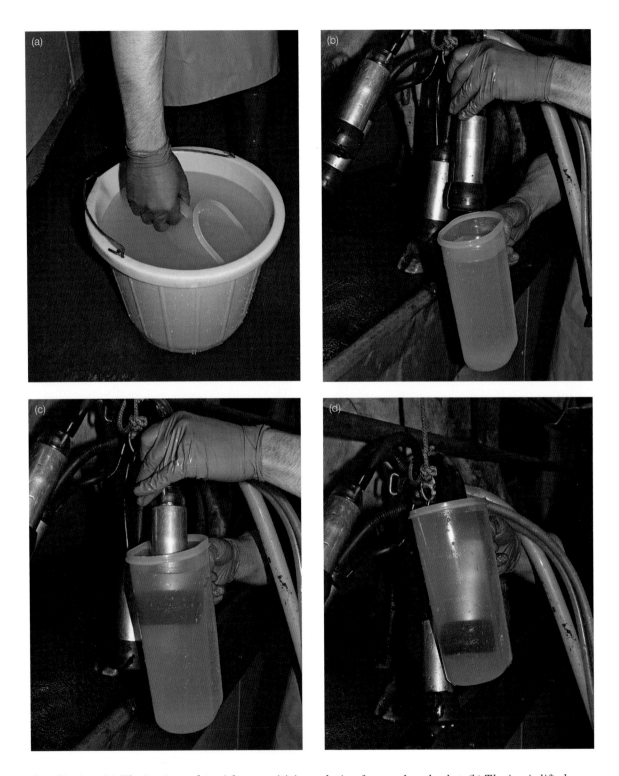

Jug dipping. (a) The jug is used to pick up sanitizing solution from a clean bucket. (b) The jug is lifted up to the liner. (c) The liner is immersed in the jug. (d) The liner is fully immersed in the jug.

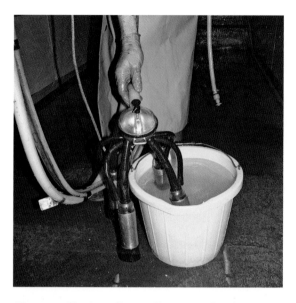

Alternate dipping: dip two liners inside a bucket while allowing two liners to remain outside the bucket .

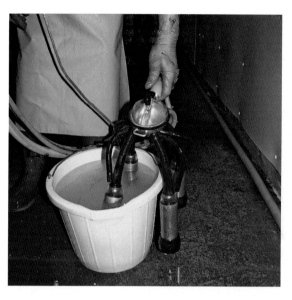

Alternate dipping – repeat the process by allowing the dipped liners to stay outside the bucket while the two undipped liners are dipped in the bucket.

flushed from the liners and, on occasions, faecal material both of which will inactivate the disinfectant. As a result, the buckets need to be changed at regular intervals, something which is probably not appreciated or performed frequently enough.

Spraying the Insides of Liners with Sanitized Water

Spraying has fewer complications but is, in practice, more complex to do and so can be more tiresome and time-consuming. Some parlours have drop lines set up specifically for the job with sanitized water, others use a household or greenhouse-type spray, which can be physically demanding. It is also possible to 'break' the long milk tube, especially if in-line filters are used and flush water or sanitized solution through the long milk tube after known infected cows. However, there can be the danger that a complicated routine for manual cluster disinfection may so occupy the time and mind of the milker that other parts of the milking routine, such as teat prep and lag time, may suffer.

Automatic Cluster Disinfection and Flushing

As with many disinfection processes, cluster disinfection can be automated. This is not a new concept and both fluid (water or sanitized

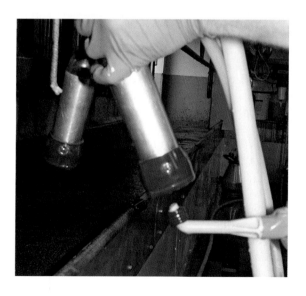

Spraying liners with a drop line.

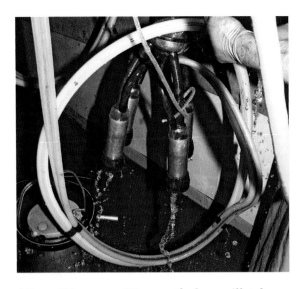

After milking a mastitis case, the long milk tube can be 'broken', especially if in-line filters are used and water or sanitizing solution is flushed through the cluster.

water) and combined (water or sanitized water and compressed air) systems have been available around the world for many years. Water-only systems were not uncommon in larger units in the USA and Israel ten to fifteen years ago. It has been suggested that the combined compressed air systems improve milk yield by reducing milk wastage or that the disinfection process is improved by destroying bacteria, although the main benefit is likely to be in drying the units before the next cow is milked. There have been some parlour set-ups in the United Kingdom over the years that included a plain water flush after milking, but these generally found little favour. The quality of the water used to flush the parlour, for example, bore hole water, can impact both mastitis and bactoscan, consequently it is more common for cluster flush systems installed now to use sanitized water.

Currently there are two common automated cluster disinfection systems in the United Kingdom: ADF, as already discussed under automated PMTD, and Clusterflush. A third system, Air Wash, manufactured by Dutch Research Innovations, flushes the liners via an extra flush pipe entering the short milk tube. These systems require a pump that can

withstand the corrosive effects of the sanitizing solution (often peracetic acid) and deliver a known final concentration of generally 0.2 to 0.5 per cent; *see* photo on page 123.

Clusterflush

Clusterflush, produced by Vaccar Ltd, is a relatively new, automated, individual cluster sanitization system which cleans and disinfects the unit after every cow is milked and will help reduce cross-contamination and infection between cows in the parlour, which, in turn, will reduce the spread of mastitis via the milking machine. The system is managed by a control box and the trigger to activate the system is via the ACR and a valve box. Once the unit has been taken off, the vacuum is reapplied to the unit to sweep as much residual milk as possible from the cluster and the

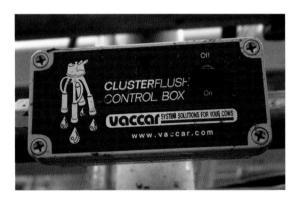

Clusterflush control box.

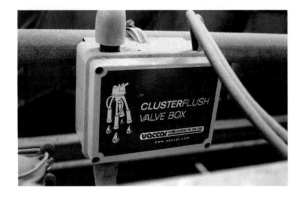

Clusterflush valve box.

long milk tube. Plain water or, ideally, sanitized water, commonly containing peracetic acid, is delivered through the long milk tube via a Y-junction to the cluster and exits via the liners. The cycle is completed by drying both the long milk tube and the cluster by blasting compressed air through to force out the water or sanitizing solution. The first flush has a degree of milk contamination, despite the initial vacuum sweep, and so a second flush and compressed air drying blast complete the process. The total time taken from cluster removal is approximately 30sec and so has little impact on the milking routine or the total time to milk a herd. The total volume of sanitized solution used per unit per cow seems to be quite variable in parlours seen by the author and ranges from 350ml (2×175 ml) through 500ml (2×250ml) to the manufacturer's recommendation of 700ml (2×350ml). These volumes are significant in terms of flushing effectiveness, and the fact that the system is flushing the long milk tube and, more critically, the cluster, including the clawpiece bowl and liners, should ensure the removal of much of the bacterial contamination from residual milk. As the system can be triggered manually, by a button on the control pad, the flush can be repeated to further improve flushing and disinfection for known mastitic or high SCC cows. The current capital outlay is approximately £500 per unit.

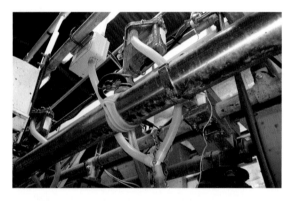

Clusterflush Y-junction plumbed into the long milk tube.

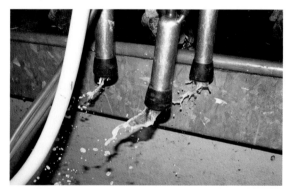

Clusterflush second and final flush.

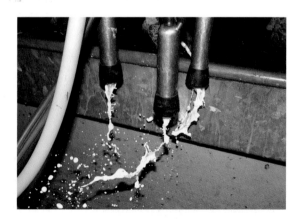

Clusterflush first flush – note the significant milk residue.

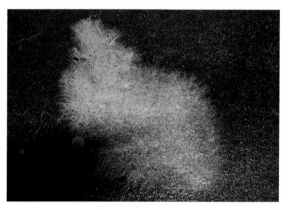

Clusterflush – flush volume from one shell with 50p coin for comparison.

Automatic Disinfection and Flushing (ADF)

ADF is discussed in detail under automated PMTD. It is a relatively new system but clearly relies on bespoke liners (with a small valve to deliver the teat disinfectant and sanitizing solution), which may have consequences when trying to fit these liners and shells to a variety of milking systems (*see* photos on pages 120–121). Early installations tended to have plain water flush systems after the delivery of the teat dip disinfectant and many continue to do so. More recent installations have incorporated a peracetic acid flush, which should give a superior performance in rapid disinfection of the liners. The delivery of the sanitizing solution through the nozzle near the liner mouthpiece will remove residual milk at the mouthpiece (and potential residues of teat dip solution), sanitize the mouthpiece and, as it is delivered by alternate flush solution under pressure followed by compressed air, to a certain extent the liner further away from the mouthpiece. The cluster is suspended on the ACR cord, with the shells hanging vertically at the time of the flushing process, so any residual milk in the clawpiece and, less significantly, the long milk tube will be relatively unaffected. ADF additionally automates the application of post-milking teat disinfection unlike Clusterflush. Current costs are approximately £1,000 per unit.

AMS ROBOTIC MILKING

Automatic milking system (AMS) or robotic milking is a relatively new technology which, despite gaining in popularity in recent years, is still in the minority. As automation of cluster removal and then cluster attachment became a reality, AMS technology was also becoming a reality. The first patents were granted in the early 1970s with the first prototypes on farms around 1985, but they were not really on commercial farms until the 1990s. Even then, initial teething problems meant that the numbers did not increase significantly until late 1990s and early in this century. A lack of available staff on farms, combined with a wish for a change in lifestyle, has made an automated, less labour-intensive approach to milking cows more attractive to some farmers since this improvement in lifestyle gives more time for family and leisure activities. The reduction in physical work could also be attractive, particularly to older farmers or those with physical health problems, which has some relevance as the average age of a dairy farmer in the United Kingdom is around fifty-five. There may also be increased opportunities for attracting and keeping skilled labour with the potential for increased profitability based on increased milk production potential and lower labour costs. AMS has the potential to offer improved udder health, as cows have 'milking on demand', with possible associated improvements in welfare. However, there are also concerns regarding the ability for AMS to accurately diagnose mastitis (*see* page 97) and that, if not correctly set up, the lack of human presence could result in the opposite effect. Research shows that the success of AMS is as much to do with the farmer's attitude and expectations as it is the cow's ability to adapt to self-service milking. Cows tend to present themselves most commonly for milking every six to nine hours on average, or nearly three times a day. The main difficulty in grazing-based dairy systems is getting the cows to come in to be milked. Feed is generally the main motivator for cows to move voluntarily into the automatic milking installation and pasture management is the key to being successful in an extensively grazed herd situation in the United Kingdom. Studies in New Zealand have used access to drinking water to help to train cows to leave their grazing area and come in to be milked.

Clearly, for AMS to be widely adopted by dairy farmers there will be a need to get used to not having the tie of milking the cows fourteen times a week and using the time saved for monitoring the robot, milk production and udder and cow health. This will also mean that a degree of computer literacy will be needed, something not all older farmers have. As with

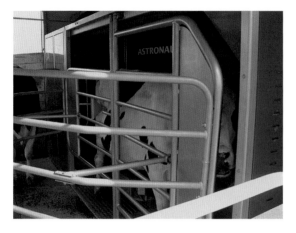

Robot or automatic milking system (AMS) crate.

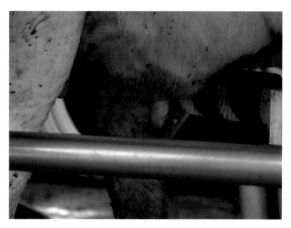

AMS milking teat preparation.

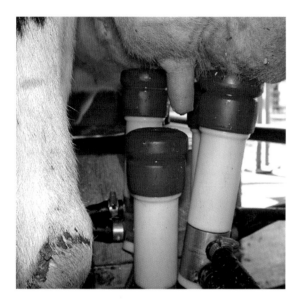

AMS unit attachment.

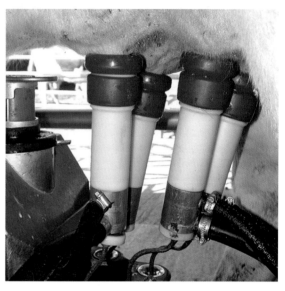

AMS milking.

all machines, AMS can break down and, since they are more complicated than the average parlour, there will also be a need for a network of on-call, skilled engineers able to deal with both hardware and software problems.

HOUSING AND ITS INFLUENCE ON MASTITIS

The likelihood of a new intramammary infection becoming established, like any other infectious disease, is a balance between the infectious agent itself, the host and the environment. The influence of the infection agent will depend upon many factors, including virulence (infectivity) and dose, while the host effect will depend upon the innate and/or acquired immunity as well as physical barriers. The environmental influences specifically in the case of mastitis will include ambient temperature, humidity, hygiene, the space available for each cow, comfort and ventilation. Many of these environmental factors will vary according to housing size (stocking density),

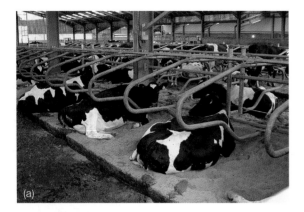

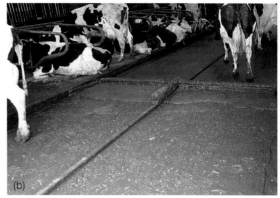

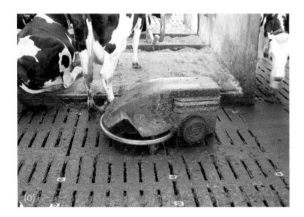

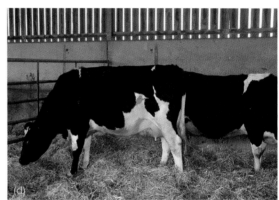

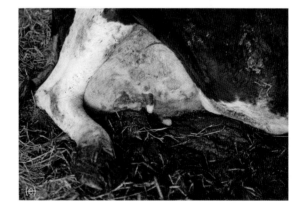

Housing is important. (a) Cow comfort. (b) Automatic scraper. (c) Robot scraper. (d) Clean straw. (e) Dirty bedding.

ventilation, housing type and, for example, bedding type. Generally, an inert bedding such as sand, will not support the growth of bacteria as it does not contain organic matter, unlike more common bedding types such as straw, wood shavings and recycled paper. Indirect measures of housing cleanliness would include visual cow hygiene (flank) scoring and, more specifically, teat hygiene scoring, which can also be performed after teat preparation and used as a measure of teat preparation efficiency. The design and

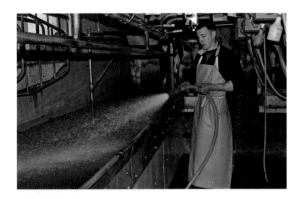

Washing the parlour to keep things clean.

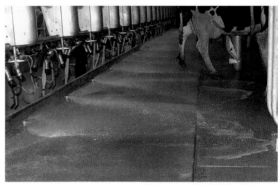

Automatic wash down after each batch of cows has been milked.

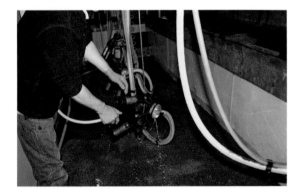

To wash units repeatedly during milking is important as they commonly become soiled during the milking.

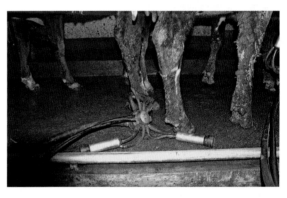

Units can be kicked off, which increases the chance of the faecal contamination of milk.

management of cow housing is critical to overall disease management and not just mastitis management. Design and the management of cubicles or straw yards, for instance, can greatly influence milk quality and mastitis rates, and guidance and information on cow housing can be found in many reference books, websites or from agricultural advisory bodies.

GENERAL HYGIENE AT MILKING TIME

General hygiene standards during milking are critical and repeated washing of the parlour in general and the cow standing and clusters in particular is essential to maintain milk quality, as well as reduce the chance of intramammary infections.

CHAPTER FIVE

Mastitis Records and Their Use

MASTITIS RECORDS AND TARGETS

Records

Farm records relevant to mastitis will be variably available, with some being a legal requirement while others are voluntary, and some having a cost such as an individual cow SCC.

Bulk Milk Somatic Cell Count (BMSCC)

All farms legally have to be sampled four or five times in a month and these data are used to calculate a monthly figure which is then used to calculate a geometric three-month mean. Geometric means tend to smooth out any atypical, 'rogue' high results and are calculated by converting the SCC to a logarithm, averaging the logarithm and then converting the result back to a number. BMSCC can also be looked at over a longer period and a twelve-month rolling mean can be a useful figure to give longer-term trends.

Clinical Mastitis Case Records

Accurate clinical mastitis records give a true record of case incidence (number of quarter treatments) and mastitis rate (cases per 100 cows). Details such as cow identity, quarter affected and treatment used, with ideally a response to treatment, will make the records more useful, and repeat and recurrence rates can then be calculated. The recurrence rate is the proportion of cases requiring one or more repeat treatments and relates to the presence of chronic infections, particularly if contagious pathogens are considered. The repeat rate includes all repeat treatments and can give an indication of the duration of existing infections and treatment efficacy, but it is significantly affected by the culling policy, that

Reference	Date	BF	UREA	PRT	SCC	BAC	ANT	
Torridge Vale Ltd.				Lab Report			Page	9
	07/02/2006	3.730 ?	0.043	3.190	161.000	47.000		517.000
	15/02/2006	3.700 ?	0.051	3.160	265.000 ?	35.000		520.000
		3.720	0.047	3.180	220.350	47.000	0.000	518.500

Individual farm bulk milk quality report from first-time buyer showing date of sampling, butterfat, urea, protein, SCC, Bactoscan, potential antibiotic violations and volume collected.

is, how many repeats are allowed before the cow is culled?

Records may be on paper or individual cow record cards, or increasingly they are recorded on a farm or veterinary practice-based computer systems such as Interherd, 1-Stop or Uniform Agri. Some web-based recording systems are being developed for farm health recording, such as CIS and FarmWizard from Northern Ireland.

Tubes Used/Purchased

All farms should have records of total lactating and dry cow tubes purchased, even if these have to be acquired from veterinary practice invoices. However, these do have limitations as the number of tubes used per mastitis case may vary and not give an accurate indication of the number of mastitis cases treated. With dry cow therapy, not all cows may be treated and the use of the internal teat seal (Orbeseal),

Health: Animal Cell Counts												NMR
Herd No.										Recording Date		
ANIMAL		LACT		Mastitis Cases -Nr -Last Case	PREVIOUS TESTS					CURRENT TEST		FARM USE
Name	Line	No.	Days		Lact Ave.	No > 200	18 JAN	22 FEB	24 MAR	24 APR	% Contrib To Herd	
ANIMALS WITH LATEST TEST 200,000 OR ABOVE												
S L DEBBIE 118	0541	1	212		254	3	179	102	81	955 +	1	
S JELT MYRTLE 44	0671	2	30		955	1				955 +	1	
S BLACKBEAUTY 17	2020	11	325		745	10	802	589	1196	793 ++		
S MANAT JEAN 207	0948	1	93		620	2		445		769 +	1	
S SARGENT BARBARA 25	0203	3	281		280	8	497	240	280	766 ++		
S CRACKER DEBBIE 139	0931	1	49		409	1			62	710 +	1	
SANDYRIDGE AGATHA 47	2410	4	219		152	1	60	82	88	695 +	1	
S PRINCIPAL JEAN 178	0369	3	14		694	1				694 +	1	
S R AARON RUBY 29	0048	3	275		136	1	72	124	43	686 +	1	
S ROYSTON AGATHA 65	0596	1	261		236	4	186	163	239	669 ++	1	
S JOCKO BARBARA 36	0731	1	250		148	1	90	39	78	669 +	1	
S FATAL DEBBIE 106	0189	2	315		176	2	150	56	573	663 ++		
S SNOWDROP 80	2090	9	161	1 23 Feb	1102	3	91	5274	549	635 ++		
S PAULA 46	2302	6	558	1 14 Jan	384	11	435	352	527	618 ++		
S PRINCIPAL RUBY 35	0343	3	180		234	3	33	213	152	599 +	1	
S L DROP JEAN 198	0832	1	46		374	1			95	599 +	1	
S P AGATHA 64	0569	2	59		312	1			82	587 +	1	
S RAPTURE JEAN 138	2479	4	342		585	5	5354	133	1164	582 ++		
S LUCENTE JEAN 200	0893	1	30		576	1				576 +	1	
879 S M DEBBIE 136	0879	1	30		559	1				559 +	1	
S ROYSTON DEBBIE 117	0516	2	189		245	2	89	117	96	557 +		
S HELEN 60	2094	10	260		175	4	107	284	288	557 ++		
SANDYRIDGE JEAN 108	2241	7	450		191	5	235	103	1311	555 ++		
S JEAN 136	2445	5	193		522	6	689	99	586	529 ++	1	
S ASTRE BLACKBIRD 89	2547	4	69		775	3		1444	685	526 ++	1	

NOTES: A cell count of "9999" means the test result was 10 million cells/ml or greater

' +' means the result was over 200,000 this month, but not last
'++' means the last two months were both over 200,000

Health: Animal Cell Counts   Version: 2.22   Date Printed:

Example of an individual cow SCC record sheet.

either as an alternative or in combination, is a complicating factor.

Sub-clinical Mastitis Records: Individual Cow SCC

SCC records give an indication of the numbers and the details of cows with sub-clinical mastitis. *See* photo on page 134 and the SCC section for details.

Bacteriological Laboratory Sample Results

Milk sample results from clinical cases, sub-clinical cases (cows with high SCC) and bulk tank (including differential TBC) may be available. Generally, the results need to be interpreted by a veterinary surgeon in conjunction with the herd history.

Milking Machine Service

Milking machine service reports can indicate the frequency of servicing and the date of the last service. Liner change intervals can be checked, with the ideal interval being 2,500 milkings for standard butyl rubber liners.

Targets

See tables below and overleaf.

QUALITY MILK PRODUCTION

Current and Historic Milk Quality Measures

Ever improving standards of hygiene in food production have been mirrored in milk production and bacterial counts in the form of TBC were introduced for payment purposes in October 1982 by the Milk Marketing Board (MMB), which, at that time, was purchasing all the milk sold in England and Wales. A carrot-and-tick method of 'encouragement' was used (as it was with SCC) to drive improvements, and the price of milk was adjusted, either as a bonus or a penalty according, initially, to the TBC and, more recently and to this day, according to the bactoscan. The TBC results were made available to all farmers producing milk for human consumption for the four months leading up to the start of the payment scheme in October 1982, and the number of herds in the top (best) band for TBC rose from one-quarter to nearly two-thirds during this time.

But it was not until after the deregulation of the national milk market on 1 November 1994 that the bactoscan method gradually superseded TBC for monitoring milk quality.

Sub-clinical mastitis targets

Parameter	Target	Interference
BMSCC ×1,000 cells/ml	<100	150
Bactoscan ×1,000 cells/ml	<20	30
No. of heifers with SCC >200,000 cells/ml	<5%	10%
No. of 2nd lactation and older with SCC >200,000 cells/ml	<10%	20%
No. of Apparent New Sub-clinical Infections (ANSI or New)	<5%	10%
No. of cows calving with 1st SCC recording >200,000 cells/ml (First)	<15%	25%

Clinical mastitis targets

Parameter	Target	Interference
Mastitis rate (cases per 100 cows)	30	40
% herd affected	20%	30%
% recurrence rate	<10%	15%
Tubes per cow in herd per year	1.5	2.5
Tubes per case	4	6
Cull rate for mastitis	<2%	5%
Dry cow mastitis (summer mastitis)	<1%	5%

As a result of this deregulation of the industry, raw milk was now being purchased direct from farms by a number of first-time buyers. Bactoscan was introduced by individual companies and used for testing for payment purposes over a period from 1995 to 1997. Most countries in Europe now use bactoscan, despite there being no limit set for the rejection of milk for human consumption, unlike the TBC, where a figure of 100,000 cells/ml is set in EU law. Farmers are paid a differential price, depending on the bactoscan level in the milk they supply. Generally, this is calculated on a two-monthly geometric mean.

Measurement of Hygienic Milk Production

TBC/TVC

Food and food products, including dairy products such as milk, cheese and yoghurt, can be easily monitored by measuring total bacterial counts (TBC), say, per gram or per ml, as appropriate. In the past, the TBC was used as a measure of milk hygiene, and payment penalty systems were applied to encourage hygienic milk production. However, because this type of measurement involves culturing live bacteria to obtain a count, the term total viable count (TVC) is used more commonly in the food industry and would, in fact, be a more appropriate term with regard to milk. The bacterial culture type of monitoring, such as TBC/TVC, is very time-consuming, taking days, not minutes, and is affected by certain types of bacterium, such as anaerobes and psychrotrophs, not growing and bacterial clumping where the bacterial numbers are underestimated. A differential TBC, in which the several sources of bacteria in milk can be estimated, is discussed in the section on bulk milk in the bacteriological culture chapter.

Bactoscan

This is a more rapid system taking minutes where all living cells are counted and do not need to be able to grow on agar under normal laboratory conditions to be counted. Anaerobes and psychrotrophs are therefore counted more accurately and there are also fewer issues with clumping, so the counts tend to be higher and more representative of the true bacterial numbers.

E. coli Count

The Food Standards Agency (FSA) always has to look at improving food safety issues and there have been suggestions that a total *E. coli* count might be introduced with a payment penalty system for raw milk supply. The suggestion is that this is with a view to reducing the risk of *E. coli* O157 which, while the prevalence in cattle is thought to be low and the bulk of milk consumed is being pasteurized, would fit well with the FSA approach to risk of the precautionary principle.

Somatic Cell Count (SCC)

What Is It and What Does It Mean?

Somatic is derived from the Greek word *somatikos* and means 'of the body'. Around

95 per cent of somatic cells are leucocytes (white blood cells), with the remainder being mainly epithelial cells, which are intermittently sloughed and shed into the milk. Both the overall absolute number and proportion of the various types of leucocyte in milk will vary with a number of factors, including stage of lactation, time of year, diurnal variation, milking frequency and interval and stress, but with the most significant changes being seen in response to infection.

Response to infection can cause variation in SCC in:

Absolute number   In the 'real', commercial world (as opposed to that of research) the use of SCC to determine udder health is generally at the cow level and is measured by using as a commingled composite samples of milk from all four quarters. However, the measurement of SCC at an individual quarter level is more appropriate in discussing the effects of infection on milk SCC and determining a threshold level above which infection is likely. It is widely accepted that milk from an uninfected gland will almost always have an SCC <100,000 cells/ml, whereas milk with an SCC >200,000 cells/ml may well indicate that it comes from an infected gland. In addition to this, there is some evidence that a very low SCC may increase the risk of intrammamry infection, and so somatic cells may offer some protection to intrammmary infection as well as being an indicator that it is present.

Proportion   The majority of somatic cells in normal bovine milk are macrophages (65 to 85 per cent), with other leucocytes, including lymphocytes (10 to 25 per cent) and neutrophils (0 to 10 per cent), making up the numbers, along with epithelial cells (0 to 5 per cent). Milk from an infected gland, however, has in excess of 90 per cent neutrophils, with an unchanged proportion of epithelial cells and macrophages and lymphocytes making up the numbers.

SCC is expressed as a number of somatic cells per ml of milk and can logically be used as an indirect measure or indicator of udder health (with the caveat that factors other than infection can affect SCC), because the majority of the SCC is made up of immune cells which are produced in greater numbers by an infected gland. For these reasons, changes in SCC are used as a proxy measure for infection.

Financial Implications

The implications and financial impact of increased SCC in terms of reduced yield and quality have never really been heeded by farmers, and it was only when the financial penalties became more direct by reduced milk value by way of a payment penalty that interest was focused on cell counts. *See* for further information the section on economics in Chapter 1.

How Is It Measured?

The simplest form of SCC measurement is done by looking down a microscope and counting (direct microscope cell count), which is very time-consuming and clearly not practicable for the high throughputs needed by the dairy industry. Automation was initially introduced by a Coulter counter, which counted the particles above a fixed size; this, however, may have included epithelial cells, cell fragments and possibly gas bubbles. When the dairy industry changed to Foss, the current method, a slight reduction in BMSCCs was seen. Most SCC measurements around the world are by the Foss technique, using a fluoro-optical principle which detects and counts cells by means of their fluorescence rather than by utilizing the particle size. This improved accuracy is because the fluorescent dye ethidium bromide penetrates the leucocyte cell wall and forms a complex with the nuclear material DNA.

Factors Affecting SCCs

Mastitis – type of bacterium   Major pathogens will tend to result in more significant SCC increases and are likely to be >200,000 cells/ml. Minor pathogens may result in insignificant SCC increases of 50,000 cells/ml or less, which may be difficult to detect and particularly at the cow level (composite sample).

Milking frequency Generally the BMSCC will be lower in herds milking three times daily when compared with twice daily, although there may be a transient increase in BMSCC when herds switch from twice to three times a day milking.

Milking interval Longer milking intervals tend to give a lower SCC, due partly to back pressure reducing cell diapedesis and partly to the increased absolute yield with a longer inter-milking interval, resulting in a greater dilution of somatic cells present; thus morning milking tends to have a lower SCC than evening milking. This became significant in the United Kingdom, with some milk recording companies using 'factoring', where milk from one milking (either morning or evening) rather than a mixture of milk from both milkings is analysed to produce monthly milk recording data. Yield, butterfat and protein can be adjusted (factored) so that the daily figures can be calculated, but this is not possible for SCC. As part of the factoring process alternate a.m. and p.m. milkings were used in consecutive months to even out protein, butterfat and yield and, as a consequence, there were significant changes in SCC at both the herd (BMSCC) but, more importantly, at the cow level, where new infection and recovery rates were distorted by these diurnal fluctuations, rather than by changes in the cow's SCC.

Seasonal variation Such variation, in the form of a summer rise in BMSCC, is seen unrelated to the stage of lactation rise observed in late lactation in seasonal calving herds. The mechanism is unclear, but is observed in many countries around the world. With the advent of climate change, some of the increase in BMSCC seen in the summer may be due to heat stress, particularly when cows are seen huddled in groups or under trees in the height of summer.

Diurnal variation The SCC is highest in the foremilk. Just after milking for several hours, it then gradually falls to the lowest level, which occurs immediately before the following milking.

Stage of lactation The SCC is elevated immediately after calving, irrespective of whether the cow is infected or not; this may, particularly in heifers, be stress related. This elevation in SCC can last up to two weeks and consequently elevated SCCs in this period must be interpreted with caution. SCCs, having fallen after this initial, elevated period in some cows, tend to rise throughout the remainder of the lactation. This is probably not primarily a physiological phenomenon but, instead, may indicate a combination of increased exposure to and acquisition of sub-clinical infections with reduced yields, resulting in reduced dilution of somatic cells particularly just before drying off. Some work has shown that these rises in the SCC in late lactation are more significant in cows with sub-clinical infections and as many cows can remain under 50,000 cells/ml right up to drying off; the excuse used for rising BMSCC in seasonal calving herds, when much of the herd is approaching drying off, may be overplayed. Perhaps it indicates a higher prevalence of sub-clinical infection than would be detected earlier in the season when most of the herd was producing more milk and the somatic cells were being diluted.

Age (more strictly, parity number) Although age is often cited as a factor in the likelihood of a cow having an elevated SCC, this is more an indication of an increased chance of its having picked up an intramammary infection and is effectively a proxy measure of exposure. In essence, older cows are more likely to have acquired an intramammary infection just by the fact that they have been milked more times, but this is nothing to do with age per se. Many old cows do have a low SCC.

Stress This can increase the SCC, although often it is difficult to be sure that other factors are not involved. Stress induced by the mixing of cows in new groups, isolating individual cows in a paddock or chasing them with a dog has been shown to increase the SCC, and it seems that the greatest increases are found in cows with a previous history of mastitis. Some preliminary work with a large database of routine monthly milk recording data has shown a possible association between low milk proteins, which might indicate nutritional stress in terms of low dietary energy, and increased SCC.

Day-to-day As with any biological system, there will be small but sometimes significant day-to-day variations in SCC. One must also remember that cows are continually doing battle with invading bacteria and winning. To achieve this, they will on occasions need to recruit large numbers of somatic cells to win the fight. If an SCC measurement is taken at that time a very high result may be recorded, which might have been considerably lower or even normal if taken some hours or days later. Cows have 'bad hair days' and one must be aware that there may be little significance of a single, high SCC result. However, if it is the beginning of a persistent infection it will, of course, be significant.

What Milk Can Be Measured?

The SCC may be measured at various stages of the production of milk for human consumption from the bulked up milk from several farms in a silo at a milk factory, through a bulk milk tank on farm, an individual cow sample, to an individual quarter sample. They will each have their own characteristics in terms of what they indicate, the significance of changes in results and their sensitivities in detecting infection. In general, the amount that a result will vary from test to test and the sensitivity of detecting infection will increase as one moves from a twelve-month rolling mean to a three-month geometric mean for farm bulk tank milk, through individual monthly and then weekly results for farm bulk tank, down to individual cow and then individual quarter samples.

Herd or Bulk Milk Somatic Cell Counts (BMSCC)

A herd or bulk milk tank SCC is effectively made up of the SCCs of the individual cows contributing milk to the bulk tank at that time. It gives an estimation of how widespread infection is (prevalence) within those cows. Although the impact an individual cow

has on the BMSCC will depend on a combination of her yield and the SCC, it can be estimated that there is an increase in prevalence of 10 per cent for every 100,000 cells/ml increase in the BMSCC. Every farm producing milk for human consumption has to have four or five 'weekly' bulk tank samples each month, which are often sent to the farmer by text message. From these results a monthly BMSCC figure is calculated, which is used to calculate a rolling three-month BMSCC geometric mean which, in turn, is used for quality payment purposes. The three-month geometric mean is calculated by converting the monthly figures to logarithms, averaging them and then using an antilogarithm to convert it back to a recognizable SCC. The effect of this is to damp down the effect of a rogue single high BMSCC, thus smoothing the figure used that farmers are paid on. Although not used for payment purposes, the rolling twelve-month average BMSCC may be a useful figure to look at for longer-term trends and for monitoring progress within mastitis health planning.

It is worth noting that the BMSCC only gives a result for the cows currently having their milk added to the bulk milk tank. Clearly, this will not include any cows currently dry nor will it include cows whose milk is being withheld from the bulk tank. These might include cows under treatment, cows freshly calved and those with a high SCC. This means that the BMSCC of milk being sold from a dairy herd (from the cows that have their milk allowed in the bulk tank) is a 'manipulated figure' and will often underestimate the herd BMSCC and thus will not reflect the true mammary health status of the herd. For those herds that do regular monthly individual cow milk recording, a better figure to use is the calculated BMSCC since usually all cows currently in milk are milk-recorded even if their milk is being withheld from the bulk tank. By calculating the theoretical BMSCC by using the yields and SCC of each cow a more realistic BMSCC is obtained, giving a truer picture of udder health status for the herd.

Individual Cow Somatic Cell Counts (ICSCC)

Regular monthly individual cow recording is probably the most common use of somatic cell counting and is almost exclusively performed on a composite commingled milk sample from all four quarters. This does introduce complications in interpreting the results as it represents the average of all four quarters (assuming all quarters are of equal yield). There is a danger that cows with infected quarters may go undetected, particularly if they have only one infected quarter with the other three having low SCCs. For example, a cow with an SCC of 180,000 cell/ml, which is below the 200,000 cells/ml threshold (most dairy farmers would be happy to have a herd of cows like that), could have three quarters with an SCC of 50,000 cells/ml and one of 570,000 cells/ml [(50 × 3) + (570) = 720, which divided by 4 = 180].

This should not be a cause for surprise or worry, it merely serves to highlight the limitations of overly interpreting individual cow SCCs. It is generally accepted that the sensitivity and specificity (that is, saying a cow is infected when it is and saying a cow is not infected when it is not) is about 75 per cent. Or, put another way, 75 per cent of cows with an infection have an SCC >200,000 cells/ml and 75 per cent of cows with an SCC <200,000 are uninfected.

The increased cost and practical issues of collecting four times as many samples make regular monthly individual quarter SCC testing really only viable for research projects. However, composite samples can be used as an indicator for further testing at a quarter level using cow-side methods such as CMT.

Interpretation After taking the many factors which influence SCC into account, it can be seen that they are only a guide to infection status. Any decisions relating to the infection status based on SCC should be based on multiple results. As with any test, when assessing infection status, repeat result and trends can increase certainty. Lactation averages, often used on lactation certificates when cows are sold, however, can be very misleading unless they are low (*see* diagram opposite). A much more useful indicator of infection status comprises the last three SCC results as it is the current infection status we are interested in and not a previous, cleared infection increasing the lactation average, or, worse still, a cow dried off with a recently acquired infection but with a sufficient number of low SCC recordings earlier in the lactation to keep the lactation average low.

Changing the SCC threshold The 200,000 cells/ml is a good general working threshold. However, with a sensitivity and specificity of 75 per cent it can be improved upon, depending on what one is trying to achieve. In common with many tests, changing the threshold to improve sensitivity will be at the expense of specificity and vice versa. However, if it is important to be more certain that cows are infected, for instance, if they were to be selected for sampling or treatment, the threshold could be raised to 300,00 cells/ml (*see* Herd Companion below). If the converse is a high priority and there is a need to be sure that cows are not infected, say, for running a 'clean' low SCC group or if an 'either/or' dry cow policy were used with antibiotic dry cow tubes for infected cows and teat seal for uninfected cows, the threshold could be lowered to 150,000 cells/ml or even 100,000 cells/ml. This would ensure that, if a misidentification occurred, it would more likely be an uninfected cow was labelled as infected. In

Comparison of quarter SCC for two cows with the same composite (commingled) cow SCC

Likely infection status	Quarter cell counts				Composite SCC (cow)
	FL	FR	BL	BR	
Infected cow	50	50	50	570	180
Uninfected cow	180	180	180	180	180

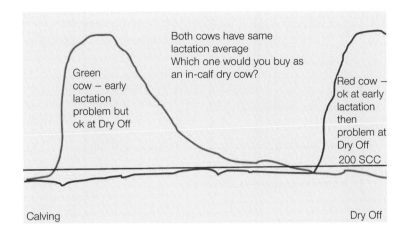

Green cow – early lactation problem but ok at Dry Off

Both cows have same lactation average Which one would you buy as an in-calf dry cow?

Red cow – ok at early lactation then problem at Dry Off

200 SCC

Calving

Dry Off

The dangers of using lactation averages to assess a cow's status (unless the average is low).

the 'clean' group scenario this might mean that an uninfected cow went into the dirty group (an error for her), but it is preferable to an infected cow going in the 'clean' group, where the error would be compounded by the spread of infection within the clean group. In the 'either/or' dry-cow approach, an uninfected cow might received an antibiotic, which is what used to happen before teat seal was developed and is better than an infected cow missing out on her best chance to be cured by being given teat seal rather than antibiotic dry cow therapy. In this latter example, it is now the case that many herds will, of course, use combination teat seal and antibiotic dry cow therapy in all cows to help prevent those which are cured during the dry period becoming reinfected just before calving.

What can individual cow SCC be used for? In common with fertility records, individual SCC records may be used in two main ways:

First, they can be used to produce action lists of cows that need to be sampled or some further action.

A second but more complex way of using individual SCC is to monitor the overall picture of changes in individual cows' SCCs in terms of new infections, recovered cows and dry-period performance, in what might be called a study of infection dynamics. As most milk recording companies have all their data on computer and the volume of milk recording data even

for one herd is considerable, various software programs have been developed to interpret infection dynamics within a herd, compare herds (benchmark) and produce action lists. One such program, Herd Companion, was developed by the author in collaboration with Drs James Hanks and Andrew James from the Veterinary Epidemiology & Economics Research Unit (VEERU), at the University of Reading, and is now available on the internet for farmers and veterinary surgeons to use at www.nmr.co.uk/ – follow the link to Herd Companion where graphs and data from a demonstration herd can be viewed and a manual downloaded. The detail and approach are discussed in the next section.

HERD COMPANION

Aim
The control and management of monthly somatic cell counts (SCC) in individual cows from recorded herds by using interpretative computer software.

Development of the Concept
Individual cow SCCs are available on a routine regular monthly basis for many herds throughout the world. In the United Kingdom individual cow cell count data became available from about 1986, and for many years since then milk recording companies have supplied farmers and vets with huge volumes

Action lists from individual cow SCC (after interpretation and not just from one result)

Action for selected problem cows	Effect on cow and/or herd
No action	Cow unaffected. Herd still at risk as infected quarter(s) still being milked through parlour*
Withhold milk (or feed to male calves)	
Treatment	Cow hopefully cured. Herd risk reduced/eliminated
Early dry off	Cow may cure
Quarter dry off/quarter culling	Herd risk reduced/eliminated†
Cull cow	Cow removed and herd risk eliminated†

*BMSCC will be reduced by 'manipulation' as the high SCC milk is not entering the tank. However, the risk of spreading infection is still present, although some form of cluster disinfection or milking last would help.

†Often by the time chronically infected cows are identified disease spread to other cows may have occurred, so even though culling will remove the infection, she will have a smug grin on her face when she is loaded on the lorry saying to herself, 'I have infected cow number 27 who will be high cell count next week and three more cows for next month.'

of paperwork which often remain within their plastic wrappers carefully filed in the farm office. Even with the advent of modern technologies, such as email and text messages, to ensure that the results get to farmers and vets rapidly, the interpretation of the data to evaluate new infection and recovery rates during lactation and the dry period has not been possible until relatively recently.

Identifying cows which cross the 200,000 cells/ml threshold, either increasing in SCC (apparent new sub-clinical infection [ANSI]) or decreasing (spontaneous – in the absence of treatment – recovery) can be monitored. Monitoring such data can not only be used to create action lists of cows needing attention, but also herd trends can be used to benchmark critical areas, such as new infection rates in lactation and dry-period performance. Regular, routine monthly analysis of individual cow SCC data can also identify cows which have recently crossed the 200,000 cells/ml infection threshold and are still infected in the following month. Identifying and treating cows

with non-recovered, new sub-clinical infections will have both direct and indirect benefits. The direct benefits will include reducing the duration of sub-clinical infections, which will, in turn, reduce the likelihood of clinical cases later in the lactation.

It might be expected that, by removing sub-clinical infections, greater milk production will ensue, but this does not often seem to be the case. Indirect benefits include a reduced prevalence of infected quarters (melting pot of infection) within the herd, which will lessen the chances of transmission, thereby resulting in a tendency to reduce the new infection rate as well. Monitoring and removing persistent new infections, where appropriate, will limit the development of chronic infections within the herd, which, in turn, will help to lower the infection pressure on other cows and may reduce the chance of clinical flare-ups within the herd. Long-term control of SCC requires an emphasis on the rapid identification of cows with raised cell counts. Close monitoring of newly infected cows can then ensure the timely treatment of those that fail to self-cure.

Both BMSCC data and monthly individual cow SCC milk recordings provide a *static* snapshot of somatic cell counts; Herd Companion emphasizes the *dynamic* nature of cell counts, and highlights the cow's changing status, not only between milk recordings but also between drying off and subsequent calving. The latter gives an indication of dry-period performance, whereas the former gives a measure of new infection and recovery rates within lactation. When using 200,000 cells/ml as a threshold infection level, one needs to take into account that the milk recording date that the data relate to bears no relation to any event dates, such as calving or drying off. Consequently, there are some limitations with data interpretation in all such regular monthly milk recording systems where cow status is determined by the SCC value. Cows with elevated SCC may have self-cured and cows with low SCC may have become infected by the time the SCC results are available (often within five to seven days). During lactation the status of a cow may be better estimated by looking at a series of results and the use of CMT can help to confirm cow status once the SCC results are available. During the dry period, estimation of infection status and dry-period performance makes the assumption that infection status will not have changed during the period between the cow's final milk recording of the lactation and actual drying off, or between calving and the cow's first recording of the next lactation, both of which could be up to four weeks. In the author's opinion this has little effect on data interpretation at the herd level.

Lactational Infection Dynamics

All cows currently in milk are allocated to one of seven status groups based on the SCC results at current and previous milk recordings. Four of the groups comprise the most likely infected cows with their latest SCC >200,000 cells/ml while, the other three groups are the most likely uninfected cows with SCC <200,000 cells/ml.

High SCC levels (>200,000 cells/ml and likely to be infected)

- *New*: not the first milk recording in the lactation but the first with a high SCC [ANSI]
- *First high*: both a high SCC and the first milk recording in a lactation
- *Repeat*: a high SCC for at least the second time in the lactation, although following a low SCC at the previous milk recording
- *Chronic*: a high SCC at both this and the previous milk recording.

Low SCC levels (<200,000 cells/ml and likely to be uninfected)

- *First low*: both a low SCC and the first milk recording in a lactation.
- *Recovered*: a low SCC level following a high SCC
- *Uninfected*: a low SCC at this and the previous milk recordings.

Where Do Today's Chronic Cows Originate from?

The author and Dr James Hanks obtained a dataset from the National Milk Records (NMR) which is a snapshot of cows recorded between 1 December 2006 and 21 January 2007. This dataset covered a total of 585,277 milking cows from 5,174 herds, which represents approximately 40 per cent of the dairy cows and herds in England and Wales (Milk Development Council, 2007). Cows with an SCC >200,000 cells/ml at the penultimate recording and the latest recording in the dataset are chronic infections based on the above definitions. Only cows that started the current lactation with a recording <200,000 cells/ml were included (lactation origin chronics), since those starting their current lactation with an SCC >200,000 cells/ml may have acquired an infection in the dry period or even in previous lactations.

Of the total cows in the dataset, 105,330 (18 per cent) had current SCCs over 200,000 cells/ml and 76,920 (13 per cent) were identified as 'chronic' high SCC cows. Of these

56,082 (10 per cent of all cows, 80 per cent of chronic cows) were deemed to be lactation-origin chronic cows. These were then traced back to find the first recording where they were >200,000 cells/ml in their current lactation. The majority (70 per cent) had an initial high SCC below 500,000, with over 50 per cent starting with SCCs below 350,000 cells/ml milk, and 24 per cent were between 200,000 and 250,000 cells/ml milk. The distributions of the latest SCC (when the data was captured) showed that 60 per cent were still <500,000 cells/ml and the peak SCC (highest SCC since the first SCC >200,000 cells/ml) had not risen >500,000 cells/ml in 36 per cent of these lactation-origin chronics.

Infection Escalator

If one assumes that cows start their milking careers with uninfected quarters (which is not always the case), the changes in the SCC once a cow is infected are quite variable. Cows acquiring an infection can be viewed as being on an infection escalator for cows, with SCCs >200,000 cells/ml where an increase in SCC results in moving up the escalator and a reduction moving down. If the SCC reduces to <200,000 cells/ml, either by self-cure (jumping off) or treatment (pushed) the cow gets off the escalator. Active SCC management utilizing interferences, such as treatment, no action or culling, must take into account the chance of success, where the selection of appropriate cows for the chosen interference is an essential part of this process. The trick is to identify cows which, if treated, could be pushed off the escalator rather than wasting time, drugs and discarded milk by treating those which are unlikely to respond.

Considerations for the Future

Accurate early identification of infection is key. As technology advances and early identification of infection becomes accurate, cow-side and available in real time, there may be significant mastitis management opportunities for early treatment. Although early treatment of any infection always gives a better chance of success, an open mind is essential when interpreting the results since treatment is likely to get the credit for all the 'self-cures'. Clearly a compromise is needed. If monitoring and identification of the causal organism of apparent, new, sub-clinical infections are followed

Cow ID	Somatic cells per 1000ml of milk	
539	2,612	
47	1,321	Where we LOOK to control somatic cell counts
272	1,302	
66	1,118	
466	1,070	
118	1,067	
396	1,061	
467	1,023	
86	992	
395	987	
248	867	
224	856	
106	848	
436	828	
26	819	
377	778	
130	685	
447	627	
474	593	
153	514	
72	503	
373	473	
380	464	
536	463	
144	441	Where most long-term somatic cell count problems BEGIN
570	437	
356	415	
333	409	
79	408	
481	397	
494	387	
219	380	
74	374	
159	374	
228	362	
524	345	
111	344	
89	339	
298	338	
407	313	
100	312	
267	310	
294	310	

Infection escalator.

through to their logical conclusion, much can be done in the prevention of infection rather than resort to treatment. However, treatment of apparent, new, sub-clinical infections (identified by culturing milk from individual quarters from cows with a rise in cell count) may be justified in certain circumstances and will help to eliminate the infections from these cows at an early stage. The decision-making process has to take many factors into account to decide if, in this instance, treatment is to be undertaken (for example, the type of pathogen involved, the number of similar SCC rises in the herd and the risk of infection spreading to other cows in the herd, cost implications with reference to cost of treatment and discarded milk versus potential financial penalties for an elevated BMSCC). Cows with a persistently elevated SCC can be considered similarly.

Advantages of Early Treatment
(This assumes that early detection is accurate and false positive diagnoses are few and rare.)

- improved welfare (mastitis is painful – even sub-clinical?)
- reduced chance of spread within the herd (most significant with contagious pathogens)
- lower production losses
- increased chance of clinical, bacteriological and cell count success.

Disadvantages of early treatment
Potentially there might be:

- treatment of cases which will self-cure
- treatment of false positive diagnoses.

Do Not Treat 'Broken' Cows
Historically, farmers and veterinarians alike have tended to concentrate on the cows with the highest SCCs as they are deemed to be 'damaging' the BMSCC most, particularly if they are high-yielding. Many of these cows will have chronic infections which are unlikely to respond to lactation therapy and should be managed (such as milked last or use of cluster disinfection) until they are either

culled or treated at drying off, when there is an increased chance of successful treatment. What is evident from this substantial dataset is that the majority of chronic SCCs begin and persist at levels that most farmers and veterinarians commonly ignore. In fact, it appears that 70 per cent of chronics start with an SCC <500,000 cells/ml and 60 per cent remain with an SCC <500,000. These chronic cows represent a major reservoir of infection in the national herd, particularly when you consider that all the SCC measurements obtained from routine milk recording reflect milk from all four quarters of the cow. Consequently, milk from a single infected quarter (cows not uncommonly have only one infected quarter) will often be considerably higher as it is diluted by milk from three uninfected quarters.

Dry-period Performance
There are four options for dry-period performance. The 200,000 cells/ml threshold is used to determine any likely changes in status, where cows can be protected, cured, acquire an infection or appear to remain infected. It is possible for this last group to include cows which are, in fact, cured during the dry period but then acquire another infection just prior to calving. This is indistinguishable from cows remaining infected throughout the dry period, because the SCC recordings are at the end of one lactation and the beginning of the next, since useful SCC measurements are only possible when cows are milking.

- *Low low*: uninfected cows remaining uninfected during the dry period
- *Low high*: cows acquiring an infection during the dry period
- *High low*: cows eliminating an infection during the dry period
- *High high*: cows remaining infected through the dry period.

Outputs from Herd Companion
It is beyond the scope of this book to cover the reports in detail, but the author has written a

guideline article: 'Getting the most from cell counts', BCVA, *Cattle Practice*, 2005, vol.13(2), pp.177–84.

Production of Monthly Action Lists

Cows with SCC >200,000 cells/ml are listed in reverse SCC in each of the four infected groups: New, First, Repeat and Chronics. The most important categories are the new and the first infections as they are recent and may justify the use of CMT to identify infected quarter(s) for sampling and/or treating. The author uses a threshold of 300,000 cells/ml within these groups when selecting cows for CMT to improve the specificity of detecting infected cows. Much extra information, such as days calved and number of recordings exceeding 200,000 cells/ml in the current and the previous lactation, are included in the reports to help with data interpretation.

The non-recovery report is probably the most important action list and lists all the cows which had a new or first infection (recent infection) in the previous month (and are still >200,000 cells/ml in the current month) with their latest SCC, so any cows still struggling with high SCCs can be identified.

Dry period details list cows calving so that those with high SCC at their first milk recording of their new lactation may be identified.

Reports with Targets and Interference Levels

Reports giving herd overviews of milk recordings, with summary data for the number of cows in the seven lactation status groups (four infected and three uninfected, based on 200,000 cells/ml SCC threshold) so, for example, the new infection rate [ANSI] (target 5 per cent of cows in milk) and first infection rate (target 15 per cent of cows calved) may be monitored.

Dry-period summary gives an indication of protection rates for cows drying off low, and cure rates for cows drying off high.

Graphs Indicating Herd Trends

There are three graphs giving an overview of herd performance:

SCC summary graphs show rolling trends for the seven lactation status groups, which allow several parameters, such as new infection rates or prevalence of chronics, to be monitored over time.

New infection graph shows the recovery rates for new infections.

Dry period graph shows an on-going view of the proportion of cows calving that are protected, cured, acquire an infection or remain infected.

The Future for Interpretive Computer Software

This software approach is making use of changes in a measure (SCC) which is used to indicate likely infection status. If future developments found a new and improved measure of intramammary infection this basic approach would still be valid. So, for example, if milk amyloid A or LDH were found to be a better measure of mammary health, the software would work equally well, with the proviso that new thresholds for change from uninfected to infected would need to be set alongside targets and interference levels.

CHAPTER SIX

Diagnosis

MASTITIS DIAGNOSIS RATHER THAN JUST DETECTION

Cow-side 'Diagnosis'

For a cow-side test to be useful it has to give an almost instantaneous result. This is a huge challenge for developers of diagnostic tests. Unless the milker can treat the cow with appropriate therapy before she is let out of the parlour, the speed at which a result is obtained becomes less critical. Most commercially available so-called 'cow-side' tests are culture-based and take in excess of 12hr, and up to 48, to get a result and so are little different in speed from a regular commercial laboratory. However, they may have a place on remote farms where sending samples to a laboratory is not convenient. These culture-based cow-side kits include Hymast, Easyculture and Petrifilm.

There are other ways of achieving a cow-side diagnosis, including the differentiation of different mastitis types by observation. Several studies have shown that the chances of a cow with a case of mastitis being systemically 'sick' or 'very sick' with reduced milk yields were greater for Gram-negative organisms (for example, *E. coli*) when compared with Gram-positive organisms (for example, *Staphylococcus aureus*). The overall accuracy of predicting the Gram-staining reaction of the organism by using milk yield and cow demeanour in these studies was approximately 78 to 79 per cent. These results show that the overall accuracy of these observations was good, and suggest that the clinical signs of cows suffering from mastitis might be useful indicators of the likely group of pathogenic organisms involved. This use of clinical indicators might allow better targeting of drug treatment type compared with the current approaches used in dairy cattle practice.

Future 'Cow-side' Diagnostic Tests

MAA milk amyloid A, as discussed in Chapter 4 on milking routine, is probably better suited to cow-side detection rather than diagnosis, although some work shows that MAA can give an indication of the causative bacteria, making it closer to diagnosis and not just detection.

PCR the polymerase chain reaction is a technique that allows the amplification (multiplying up) of genetic material, usually DNA, so that, for example, further identifying tests can be performed. PCR is a highly specific diagnostic test which could, in the future, become a cow-side test that is used in the parlour to give results in a few minutes. The technique has many applications, for example, forensics, where human DNA sequences can be used to identify and link to an individual or, in the case of bacterial or viral DNA, for rapid diagnostics. Currently the tests take hours (rather than a day or more for culturing bacteria), which is insufficiently rapid to be a cow-side test. There are also some limitations with PCR diagnostics in that it has the ability to pick up parts of DNA and so the bacterium or virus does not have to be live or even present as a whole pathogen or be present in significant numbers. This will have implications in milk samples since the presence of one or two bacteria in a sample does not necessarily indicate that the quarter was or is infected with that pathogen. PCR techniques are continuing to advance and real-time PCR (measuring the increase in DNA as it is amplified) has some ability to semi-quantitatively indicate the number of pathogens detected in the original sample.

BACTERIOLOGICAL CULTURE – THE GOLD STANDARD

Bacteria in the dairy environment can cause clinical mastitis, increased SCC or bactoscan problems. There are many different bacteria able to do this, often requiring different control measures, with obvious and significant broad-brush differences between those originating from contagious and environmental sources as well as more subtle differences in control measures for individual bacteria types. It is possible for different bacteria to influence any one, all three or a combination of clinical mastitis, increased SCC and bactoscan. As a result, to know the predominant bacteria causing a particular problem is essential if control is to be achieved. The diagnostic usefulness of milk samples cultured to determine the bacteria involved will depend on the quality of the sampling and of the sample on arrival at the laboratory. Temperature and the speed of transport to the laboratory are important. Contaminant bacteria may well mask causal pathogens and make interpretation risky, as there is no guarantee that any potential mastitis-causing bacteria originate from within the udder. Results from poorly taken, contaminated samples will indicate just that, resulting in wasted time effort and money.

TAKING MILK SAMPLES

See the accompanying box.

> **Summary of Sample Collection**
>
> - wash/dry, if needed
> - dip/wait
> - wipe
> - swab
> - strip
> - swab
> - sample

How to Take a Clean Quarter Milk Sample

Preparation

- label sterile sample bottles and fill out any forms ahead of time
- ensure hands are clean and put on a clean pair of gloves.

Clean teats

- wash teats with sanitized udder wash and dry teats with individual towels
- pre-dip, if available, and allow 30sec of contact time
- wipe off teat dip with an individual towel
- repeatedly clean and disinfect the teat end with cotton wool swabs soaked in surgical spirit or methylated spirit; repeat and discard the cotton wool swab until it appears clean strip out and discard the foremilk (five or six squirts).

Take sample

- clean and disinfect the teat end with a cotton wool swab soaked in surgical spirit or methylated spirit; if multiple quarter or a commingled composite sample is being taken from all four quarters, start with the teat furthest from you and work toward the closest teat; use a fresh swab on each teat.

- collect the milk sample by holding the sample bottle as horizontal as possible, do not allow anything to come into contact with the mouth of the bottle or the inside of the lid
- collect one or two squirts of milk from each quarter, starting with the closest quarters and working toward the ones furthest away.

Send to lab

- refrigerate samples until they reach the lab; if samples will not reach the lab within 24hr they can be frozen and kept frozen until they do reach the lab.

How to Take a Clean Bulk Milk Tank Sample

Preparation

- label sterile sample bottles and fill out any forms ahead of time
- ensure hands are clean and put on a clean pair of gloves; long, rectal examination gloves can be useful if reaching into an older type of tank to dip out the sample
- turn on the bulk tank agitator for 2min to mix the milk thoroughly.

Take sample

- older type of ice bank bulk tank
  - often has large lid covering whole tank
  - lift lid and carefully lower a sterile bottle into the milk until it fills – avoid letting go of the bottle at all costs!
- modern bulk tank
  - often has small openings in the upper surface which are not suitable for sampling
  - run milk to waste from valve used for collecting milk for a few seconds and then collect a mid-stream sample.

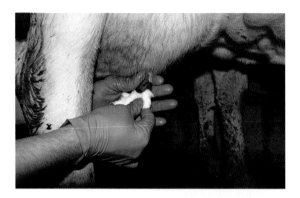
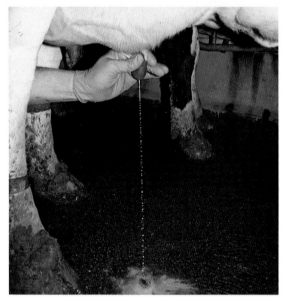
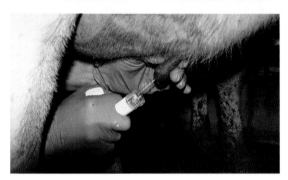

Taking a clean sample. From top to bottom: swabbing a teat end; also appropriate before administering an intramammary tube. Stripping out the foremilk; also appropriate for teat preparation. Hold the bottle nearly horizontal to prevent contaminating matter from falling into the bottle.

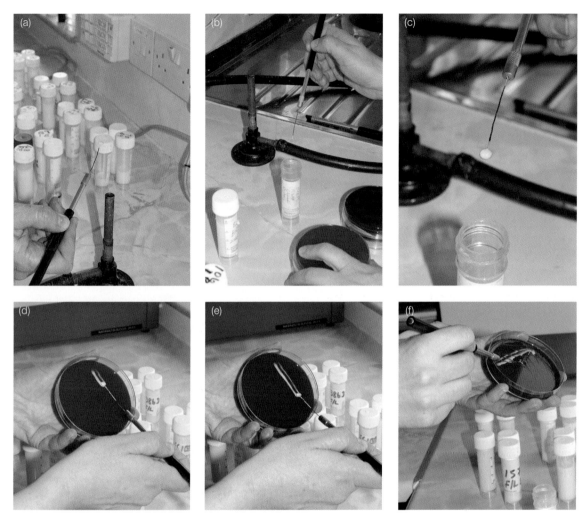

Plating up. (a) Flame loop to sterilize. (b) Platinum loop holds 3µml of milk. (c) Pick up aliquot of milk. (d) Plate on to media. (e) Spread primary innoculum. (f) Flame loop and streak out to dilute to form single colonies.

Send to lab

- refrigerate samples until posted to lab; send with coolpack or deliver to lab 'on ice'.

PLATING, INCUBATION AND IDENTIFICATION

Plating or plating up describes the transfer of a small aliquot of milk from a milk sample to a growth medium and in such a way that, when the plate is incubated, individual colonies of bacteria grow and can be identified. Milk samples frequently contain low bacterial numbers and so often increased initial inocula are used before they are streaked out to ensure that single colonies are grown, if larger numbers of bacteria are present.

The media most commonly used for mastitis bacteriology are blood agar, Edwards and McConkey media, with the additional use of Baird Parker media when *Staphylococcus aureus* is suspected. The combination of SIM media (sulphide production, indole production

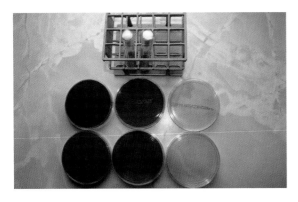

Media used in milk bacteriology: test tubes SIM media; left to right top row: Edwards media, McConkey media, Baird Parker; second row: blood agar, citrate agar and Iso-sensitest agar.

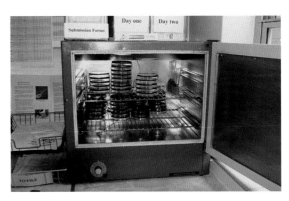

Incubator.

and motility) and Simmons citrate agar is used for the differentiation of Enterobacteriaceae. An antibiogram can be performed often on Iso-sensitest agar to determine the antibiotic sensitivity of bacterial isolates.

The plates are incubated at 37°C and then examined for growths at 24 and 48hr. The bacteria can be identified by a variety of methods, including the visual appearance of the colony on the plate and its shape, size and staining with various stains when the bacteria are viewed under a microscope.

Mastitis is almost exclusively caused by bacteria and these may be classified in many ways.

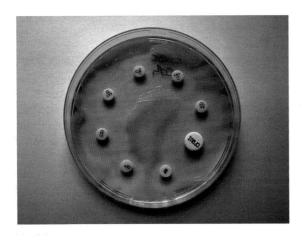

Antibiogram – antibiotic sensitivity test.

Gram-Stain

Prepare a glass slide by drying a smear of the bacteria to be tested by suspending the colony in a drop of distilled water on the slide and heat drying with a bunsen burner to fix the bacteria firmly to the slide.

1. Flood the slide with 1 per cent **crystal violet** stain and leave for 1min.
2. Wash off with gently running water and flood the slide with **Gram's iodine** and leave for 1min. [Gram's iodine is not a stain but acts a mordant to fix the crystal violet stain.]
3. Wash off with gentle running water then add a few drops of a decolorizer, such as **acetone** for a few seconds. [If the bacteria are Gram-positive they will remain 'purple' and hold the crystal violet, if they are Gram-negative the crystal violet will be removed and the slide will appear colourless.]
4. Wash off with gently running water then flood the slide with **carbol fuchsin** and leave for 1min.

[*Gram-negative bacteria will now take up the 'pink' stain while Gram-positive bacteria will remain the purple from the crystal violet.*]

5. Wash off with water and dab dry with a paper towel or allow to air dry.

View the finished slide with a microscope by using an oil immersion lens.

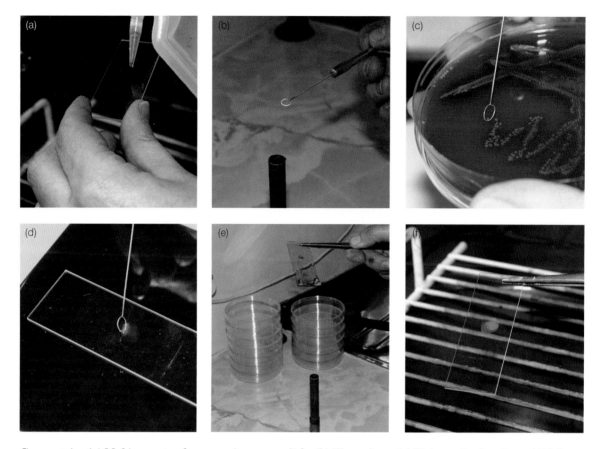

Gram-stain. (a) Making water drop on microscope slide. (b) Flame loop. (c) Pick up single colony. (d) Mix colony to emulsion in water drop. (e) Slide is dried over Bunsen burner flame to fix slide. (f) Dried smear ready for staining.

The classification can be applied at several levels and, at its simplest, may relate to the shape of the bacteria themselves; round-shaped bacteria are described as cocci, rod-shaped are described as bacilli, and bacteria with a shape somewhere in between are described as coccobacilli. Other simple methods of categorization are their differential take-up of a stain, for example, Gram-stain. The shape (cocci or bacilli) and colour (to Gram-staining) has been a fundamental part of not just mastitis bacterial identification for many years.

For the purposes of bacterial identification in mastitis the shape and use of a Gram-stain are good starting points. In general, Gram-negative (pink) rods are most often environmental in behaviour and *E. coli* would perhaps be the best known example. Gram-positive (purple) cocci are more commonly associated with a contagious mode of spread, and *Staphylococci* and *Streptococci* would fall into this category. There are no Gram-negative cocci of any note in cattle diseases, but Gram-positive bacilli do cause a variety of diseases, including mastitis, and would include *Corynebacterium* and *Bacillus* species.

Although this 'shape and colour' identification is a good starting point, further diagnostic tests are required to give a robust identification to a species level. There are a variety of confirmatory tests which generally make use of the metabolic characteristics such as the ability to ferment certain sugars (API, SIM media or Simmons citrate

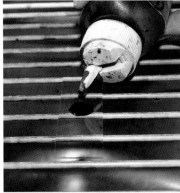

Gram-stains used.

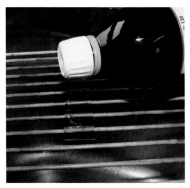

Crystal violet.

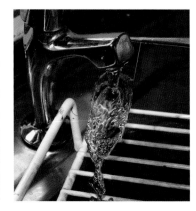

Wash slide with water.

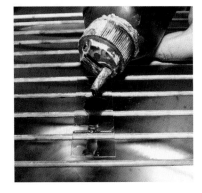

Gram's iodine.

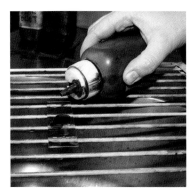

Acetone.

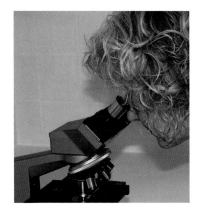

Carbol fuchsin.

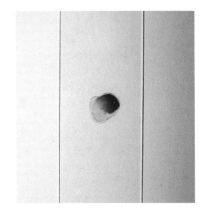

Finished slide.

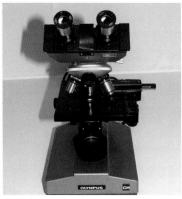

Microscope.

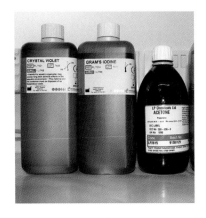

Viewing slide down microscope.

agar) or to produce certain enzymes, such as catalase or coagulase. In general, these tests require a degree of identification before their use and many are not specific to one bacterial type. For example, the catalase test will distinguish *Staphylococci* from *Streptococci*, but this relies on an identification to a Gram-positive cocci level initially

153

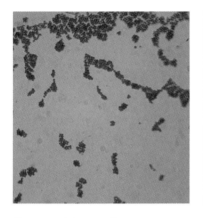

Gram-positive cocci.

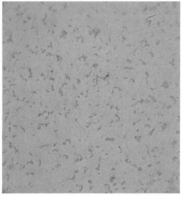

Gram-negative bacilli.

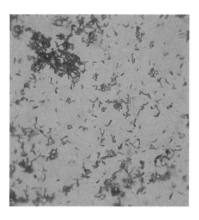

Gram-positive bacilli.

as some strains of *Bacillus* species (a Gram-positive bacillus) are also catalase producers.

INTERPRETING THE RESULTS

See also Appendix VII. In general, semi-quantitative interpretation is used and the number of colony-forming units (cfus) is taken into account. However, repeat plating out and culture of a given milk sample, even when using a standard inoculum, will give rise to variable numbers of cfus, and so interpretation must be based on trends rather than absolute numbers. Equally, the number of different types of pathogen isolated from a single sample will greatly influence the interpretation of the significance of each pathogen. Certain pathogens can be deemed to be

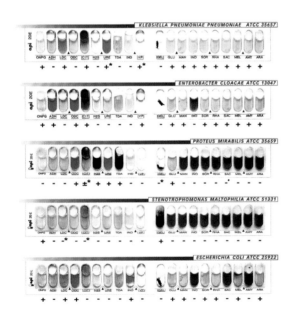

API strips can be used to distinguish various bacterial species, in this case Enterobacteriaceae.

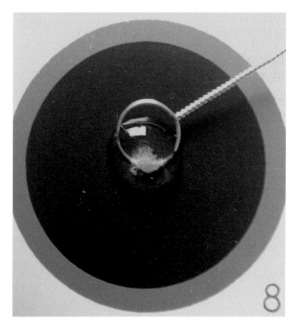

Catalase test.

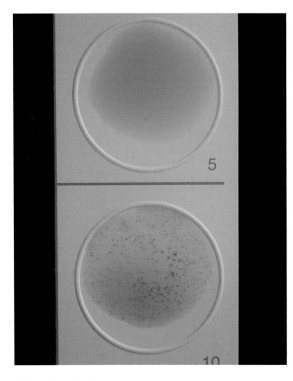

Coagulase test.

significant when isolated, irrespective of other pathogens isolated concurrently. The significance of the isolation of contagious pathogens where the major source of infection is infected quarters is generally easier to interpret. *Staphylococcus aureus* would be such an example and would always be a significant finding, indicating the presence of the pathogen in the herd, but not its prevalence. Individual cow or quarter samples would indicate infection in that cow, whereas positive culture in a bulk sample would indicate the presence of *Staphylococcus aureus* in the herd. For this reason regular bulk milk culture can be a useful tool for monitoring the presence of *Staphylococcus aureus* in a herd.

The sensitivity of bulk milk sampling to indicate the presence of *Staphylococcus aureus* in a herd is poor and so repeat sampling is advisable. Intermittent excretion, a feature of *Staphylococcus aureus* infection, may result in a false negative on single culture. The significance of the isolation of environmental pathogens where the major source is more commonly the environment is more difficult

Bacterial identification. API strips can be used to identify specific species type. Genus identification is required before the specific API strip is used

Test name	Method	Use	Pre-confirmatory test
API	After primary culture colonies are inoculated and incubated in a variety of capsules containing specific sugars different test panels are prepared in dehydrated forms which are reconstituted upon use by addition of bacterial suspensions. After incubation, positive test results are scored as a seven-digit number (profile). Identity of the bacterium is then derived from the database with the relevant cumulative profile code book or software	The use of panels with appropriate combinations of sugars allows differentiation of bacteria within groups such as Enterobacteriaceae, *Staphylococci*, *Streptococci*	Morphological examination and Gram-stain with catalase test to identify to a genus level, e.g. Enterobacteriaceae, *Staphylococci*, *Streptococci*

Additional diagnostic tests for Gram-positive cocci

Test name	Method	Use	Pre-confirmatory test
Catalase test	Add 3% hydrogen peroxide to a colony on a slide or dark tile. Catalase-positive cultures produce O_2 and bubble at once. The test should not be done on blood agar because blood itself contains catalase	Distinguish *Staphylococci* from *Streptococci*	Gram-stain to confirm Gram-positive cocci
Coagulase test	Various with varying sensitivity and specificity. Tube, slide or latex agglutination. Turbidity or clumping indicates a positive	Distinguish *Staphylococcus aureus* from coagulase-negative *Staphylococci*	Gram-stain to confirm Gram-positive cocci and catalase test positive to identify as *Staphylococci*
Lancefield Group test	Various reagents to various groups with clumping indicating a positive reaction	Used to speciate (identify at a species level) *Streptococci*	Gram-stain to confirm Gram-positive cocci and catalase test negative to identify as *Streptococci*
Edwards media (Aesculin)	The glycoside aesculin is added to a blood agar plate to give blood aesculin or Edwards plate Aesculin fluoresces under ultra-violet light, but fluorescence is lost when the glycoside is hydrolysed by aesculin-splitting bacteria to aesculetin and glucose	Distinguish between aesculin-splitting *Streptococci* (e.g. *Streptococcus uberis, Streptococcus faecalis* and *Streptococcus bovis*) and non aesculin-splitting *Streptococci* (NASC) (e.g. *Streptococcus agalactiae* and *Streptococcus dysgalactiae*	Gram-stain to confirm Gram-positive cocci and catalase test negative to identify as *Streptococci*
Baird Parker media	Colonies of *Staphylococcus aureus* are 1–1.5mm in diameter, appear black, convex and shiny. Usually surrounded by a clear zone but occasionally opaque zones will form within this clear zone. Other bacteria which may grow on this medium are easily distinguished from *Staphylococcus aureus* as they do not form black colonies	Isolate and enumerate *Staphylococcus aureus* (coagulase-positive *Staphylococci*)	Gram-stain to confirm Gram-positive cocci and catalase test positive to identify as *Staphylococci*

Additional diagnostic tests for Gram-negative bacilli

Test name	Method	Use	Pre-confirmatory test
LACTOSE FERMENTING			
The use of SIM media and Simmons citrate agar allows the following differentiation test to be performed (*see* table on page 158).			
Simmons citrate agar			
Citrate	Primary culture subcultured on to Simmons citrate agar and incubated for 48hr. Positive reaction changes the media from green to bright blue	Differentiation of Enterobacteriaceae based on the utilization of citrate as the sole source of carbon.	Morphological examination and Gram-stain to identify to a genus level of Enterobacteriaceae
SIM media – 3 tests in 1			
After primary culture a colony is inoculated by inserting a straight wire to about one third of the depth of the medium in a test tube and incubated for 18 hours or longer			
Motility	See above for method Non-motile grow only along line of inoculation. Motile show either a diffuse even growth spreading from the inoculum or turbidity of the whole medium	Differentiate various Enterobacteriaceae (*see* table on page 158)	Morphological examination and Gram-stain to identify to a genus level of Enterobacteriaceae
Hydrogen sulphide	See above for method Positive production is shown by blackening of the line of inoculation	Differentiate various Enterobacteriaceae (*see* table on page 158)	Morphological examination and Gram-stain to identify to a genus level of Enterobacteriaceae
Indole	See above for method After incubation 0.2ml of Kovac's reagent is added to the test tube and allowed to stand for 10min. Positive reaction is a dark red colour in the reagent	Differentiate various Enterobacteriaceae (*see* table on page 158)	Morphological examination and Gram-stain to identify to a genus level of Enterobacteriaceae
Further differentiation			
Oxidase	After primary culture a colony is placed on a filter paper and the reagent added. A purple colour indicates a positive reaction	Distinguish *Pseudomonas* or *Pasteurella* from other Enterobacteriaceae	Morphological examination and Gram-stain to identify to a genus level of Enterobacteriaceae
NON-LACTOSE-FERMENTING			
Further differentiation test for non-lactose-fermenting (NLF) bacteria			
Urea	Primary culture subcultured on to a urea slope. A change from pale yellow to bright pink indicates ability to 'split' urea.	Differentiate between non-lactose-fermenting (NLF) bacteria such as *Proteus* which splits urea and *Salmonella* spp. which do not, and is perhaps more used in enteric bacteriology.	Non-lactose-fermenting colony on McConkey media. Lactose-fermenting colonies appear pink on McConkey media

Look-up table for differentiation of common Gram-negative mastitis-causing bacteria

Organism	Citrate	Motility	Indole	Hydrogen sulphide	Oxidase	Lactose
E. coli	–ve	+ve	+ve	–ve	–ve	+ve
Enterobacter	+ve	+ve	–ve	–ve	–ve	+ve
Klebsiella	+ve	–ve	+ve –ve	–ve	–ve	+ve
Serratia	+ve	+ve	–ve	–ve	–ve	+ve
Pseudomonas	+ve –ve	+ve	–ve	–ve	+ve	–ve
Pasteurella	–ve	–ve	–ve	-ve	+ve	+ve
Citrobacter	+ve	+ve	+ve	+ve	–ve	+ve
Proteus	+ve –ve	+ve	+ve –ve	+ve	–ve	+ve

Key: +ve = Positive, –ve = Negative.

to interpret. *Coliforms* and *Streptococcus uberis* would be examples and the interpretation is then largely dependent on the presence of other pathogens and, in particular, the profile (both number and type) of pathogens isolated. In the case of the isolation of environmental infections the type of sample will also influence the interpretation. In a bulk sample the presence of *Coliforms*, whether in pure culture or mixed with other pathogens, would be unlikely to have any bearing on the udder health status of the cows contributing to the sample, but may well reflect the milk quality in terms of faecal contamination from dirty teats at milking. However, in a sample from a clinical mastitis case the presence of a pure and significant number of *Coliform* bacteria such as *E. coli* is highly likely to be indicative of the causal agent.

Bulk Milk Sample

Bacterial isolates from bulk milk samples are typically heterogeneous mixtures of various taxonomic and ecological groups. Theoretically, any bacterial isolate from a bulk milk sample could arise from an intramammary infection (IMI). The probability of an isolate originating from an IMI is dependent upon the bacteria. A primary function of bulk milk sample culturing is to determine whether a herd is positive for the major contagious pathogens *Staphylococcus aureus* and *Streptococcus agalactiae*. The presence of these pathogens in a bulk milk sample almost always indicates the presence of infected quarters in the herd. The presence of *Coliforms* or *Streptococcus uberis* in bulk samples is more difficult to interpret. However, on occasions the presence of *Streptococcus uberis* in large numbers in bulk samples can often be related to herds where sub-clinical infection is common or where bactoscan problems are being experienced and *Streptococcus uberis* is suspected as being part of the problem.

Composite (Commingled) Samples or Quarter Samples

Composite samples from all four quarters from one cow are also more likely to contain a heterogeneous mixture of bacteria from several taxonomic and ecological groups. However, the presence of contagious pathogens such as *Staphylococcus aureus* or *Streptococcus agalactiae* is always significant. Quarter samples

Confirmatory test for Gram-positive bacilli

Test name	Method	Use	Pre-confirmatory test
Catalase test	Add 3% hydrogen peroxide to a colony on a slide or dark tile. Catalase-positive cultures produce O_2 and bubble at once. The test should not be done on blood agar because blood itself contains catalase.	Distinguish *Corynebacterium bovis* from other *Corynebacteria*	Gram-stain to confirm Gram-positive cocci bacilli

are more likely to yield one taxonomic group, particularly in clinical cases. High cell count quarters may yield multiple taxonomic groups. Care is needed to evaluate the significance of the bacteria number and type isolated. Environmental pathogens always have the chance of being a contaminant. 'No growths' can also be problematical to interpret. In clinical samples a 'no growth' may well be as a result of the presence of Gram-negative bacteria that are non-viable and therefore unable to be cultured.

Often in clinical cases caused by Gram-negative infections the bacteria are inactivated in the udder within a few hours of infection. Milk is a 'living' medium and some of the mechanisms enabled in the udder by the cow to combat infection will continue to be active in milk, which may result in the inactivation of bacteria in the milk sample after it has been taken. In the case of clinical samples it is the released endotoxin as a result of bacterial death that causes the swelling of the quarter and, in some circumstances, systemic illness in the cow. In sub-clinical cases a 'no growth' may well be a true negative culture, but intermittent excretion of pathogens such as *Staphylococcus aureus* may result in an incorrect interpretation indicating the absence of infection. Repeat sampling and culture will help to reduce the problem of reduced sensitivity of single samples.

TYPES OF SAMPLE PROCESSED THROUGH THE AUTHOR'S MILK LABORATORY

Bulk Samples

Routine Monitoring
Samples are cultured to monitor predominant pathogens and indicate whether contagious pathogens appear to be prevalent. Interpretation includes the assessment of the presence or absence of major contagious pathogens such as *Streptococcus agalactiae* or *Staphylococcus aureus*. The semi-quantitative assessment of the presence of other pathogens can be used as a useful indicator. For example, *Coryne bovis* can be used as an indirect measure of the efficacy of post-milking teat disinfection and *Strep dysgalactiae* as an indication of teat condition, with particular reference to teat sores and blackspot. Environmental pathogens such as *E. coli*, *Coliform* or *Streptococcus uberis* are usually indicative of contamination, especially if accompanied by *Streptococcus faecalis* and *Bacillus* spp.

Differential TBC (Total Bacterial Count) or TVC (Total Viable Count)
This test is more a measure of hygienic milk production and is most commonly used in bactoscan problem investigations; however,

potential mastitis-causing bacteria will also be quantified. Although most first-time buyers of milk ex-farm use bactoscan as an indicator of production hygiene, differential TBC can give a good insight into the source of contaminant bacteria, which can originate from the milking plant and, effectively, the outside of the cow's teats as teat skin contaminants or inside the teat as mastitis bacteria. The test is effectively a TVC as it is based on culture, and so only viable bacteria are counted. It is essential that the milk arrives at the laboratory chilled and couriers and cool packs can be a disincentive to using this test. As the number of differential TBCs performed in the United Kingdom is limited, the author would suggest sending bulk milk for this purpose to the National Milk Laboratories (NML) for Bacto breakdown, to Eurofins for Mybact or to Gloucester Laboratories for bulk tank analysis, with the latter offering an experienced veterinary surgeon's interpretation of the results.

Bulk milk is cultured on different media at given temperatures with a variety of pre-culture techniques carried out to give an indication of the importance of the various sources of bacterial contamination of bulk milk, as follows:

- the total number of viable bacteria (TVC)
- thermoduric or laboratory pasteurization count (LPC) – efficacy of milking plant cleaning
- psychrotrophs – efficiency of milk cooling
- *Coliform* count – teat and cow hygiene from faecal contamination
- pseudomonads count – teat contamination from non-enteric sources
- presence of significant major or minor mastitis pathogens, for instance, *Staphylococcus aureus*, *Streptococcus asgalactiae*, *Streptococcus uberis*, coagulative-negative *Staphylococcus* and *Coryne bovis* bacterium.

Targets for each parameter may vary with the methodology and should be obtained from the laboratory.

Cow or Quarter Samples

In general quarter samples are preferable to composite samples (commingled quarter milk from more than one quarter from one cow), especially if semi-quantitative interpretation is required. Composite samples have a higher chance of being contaminated and are more difficult to interpret, especially if multiple mastitis pathogens are isolated. Composite samples do, however, have a place in reducing the costs for the screening of cows for *Staphylococcus aureus* or *Streptococcus agalactiae*, particularly when large numbers of cows are to be sampled. In general, inoculum volumes should be increased when composite samples are cultured, in an attempt to maintain test sensitivity. These composite screening sample results are then expressed as positive or negative for *Staphylococcus aureus* or *Streptococcus agalactiae*.

Samples from Individual Quarters

Clinical Mastitis Samples
A sample from an affected quarter – by definition has to be a quarter sample. Almost any bacteria isolated in pure and profuse growth can be deemed to be a possible causal agent.

Repeat Cases
A sample from affected quarter – again by definition has to be a quarter sample. Interpretation will depend on the significance of current and previous sample results. A culture of the same pathogen type will tend to indicate persistent infection, especially with Gram-positive pathogens.

Sub-clinical Mastitis Samples – High Somatic Cell Count (HSCC) Sample
Ideally, individual quarter samples – otherwise several potential causal agents may be isolated and it will not be possible to determine which quarter is infected with which pathogen. If potential environmental pathogens such as *E. coli* or *Streptococcus uberis* are isolated in mixed culture, even if with

potential contagious pathogens, it will be difficult to differentiate contamination from significant culture.

Post-treatment Check

Sample from affected quarter – again by definition has to be a quarter sample. This could be after therapy of a clinical or sub-clinical case. Culture of the same pathogen in both pre- and post-treatment samples indicates probable bacteriological treatment failure. Timing after the cessation of treatment is important. Sampling too soon after treatment will give rise to false hopes of bacteriological cure (the infection having only been suppressed not eliminated). Sampling too late after treatment may give a pessimistic measure of treatment success as reinfection may have occurred. In our practice, we tend to go for ten to fourteen days after the last tube. Intermittent excretion seen with *Staphylococcus aureus* will increase the chance of a false negative result.

Intermittent Serial Quarter Testing (ISQT)

This is used specifically for increasing the chance of isolating *Staphylococcus aureus*. It involves serial quarter sampling over a period of one week, with two frozen samples and one fresh one. ISQT may be used to increase the sensitivity of detection of *Staphylococcus aureus* in both high SCC cows and post-treatment sample checks. The three samples taken over one week help to overcome the intermittent excretion often seen with *Staphylococcus aureus*, while the frozen samples may improve the isolation of intracellular *Staphylococcus aureus* bacteria. The expansion of ice crystals during freezing causes the neutrophils to rupture and release the *Staphylococcus aureus*, increasing the chance of positive culture. This sampling regime can be combined with the use of a *Staphylococcus aureus* selective media, such as Baird Parker media, to improve sensitivity of *Staphylococcus aureus* detection.

Contaminated Samples

The definition of a contaminated sample for Veterinary Laboratories Agency (VLA) data for VIDA disease surveillance report is three types of bacterium isolated from a single sample. I would still consider *Staphylococcus aureus* to be significant in a sample where *Staphylococcus aureus*, *Streptococcus faecalis* and *E. coli* were cultured. However, *Coliform*, *Strep faecalis* and *Streptococcus uberis* could well be a contaminated sample. The presence of *Proteus* or *Bacillus* spp. would almost invariably indicate contamination of the sample. *Coliform* and contamination is a difficult area to interpret. Anecdotal evidence would suggest that many people say a 'no growth' is probably an *E. coli*, particularly in clinical mastitis, but would say that two or three colony-forming units of *E. coli* probably constitute contamination.

CHAPTER SEVEN

Treatment Options

GENERAL CONSIDERATIONS

The evolution of mastitis therapy on the farm has been considerable, from the pre-antimicrobial era, when symptomatic treatments such as massage, the use of embrocations and 'stripping out' were all that was available. The development of antimicrobial preparations for mastitis treatment heralded a new era and hopes were that mastitis would be eliminated.

The dynamics of intramammary infection is a balance between elimination (either self-cure or as a result of treatment) and the acquisition of infection, and the prevalence of infected quarters in a herd is influenced by the new infection rate and the duration of infection. Both the new infection rate and the duration of infection can be affected by:

- antimicrobial treatment, either during lactation or at drying off
- management control strategies
  - teat dipping
  - culling policy
  - milking-machine maintenance
  - general levels of hygiene.

Economic constraints and concerns about antibiotic residues have encouraged short treatment courses, with short withhold periods. This is probably contrary to the requirement of an ideal treatment protocol. The successful treatment of existing infections impacts mainly on the duration of infection, but exerts some effect on the rate of new infection by reducing the prevalence of infected quarters and therefore the level of challenge within the herd.

Mastitis control plans should include the early identification and prompt treatment of clinical mastitis, and the early identification of sub-clinical mastitis, assessment and, where appropriate, the elimination of infection either by treatment or by drying off problem quarters, the early drying off of problem cows or by culling infected cows.

The requirement for high quality milk, in particular with a low SCC, has sharpened the focus on sub-clinical mastitis. Over time, this has led to the development of various management tools to help to identify sub-clinical infections, which, in turn, has created a demand for ways to eliminate sub-clinical infections. However, one must not forget that the importance of farm protocols to prevent new infections remains. The financial penalties based on the BMSCC, levied at a producer level, have had a significant impact over recent years. The ability to finely control individual cows' cell counts, such that the BMSCC is maintained at an optimum, is becoming of paramount importance. As a result, effective and accurate early identification of infection, often by laboratory tests, the selection of specific antimicrobial therapy, again often based on laboratory tests, and the application of a specific treatment regime is becoming an important part of herd mastitis control.

As an adjunct to treatment, appropriate advice on the relevant management control measures can be given in the light of the epidemiological knowledge of the predominant bacteria involved. This will help to stop infection spreading to uninfected cows in the herd. By using this more holistic, whole-herd approach, both the new infection rate and the duration of infection are closely scrutinized.

The triggers for mastitis treatment are:

- identification of clinical mastitis should always trigger treatment
- identification of sub-clinical mastitis may trigger treatment, depending on:
  - herd BMSCC in relation to payment penalty bands
  - individual cow SCC and yield
  - previous cow history
    clinical cases
    sub-clinical cases – number and sequence of raised SCC
    other health history, e.g. lameness increasing chance of early cull.

While the treatment of clinical cases is generally seen as a given, the decision to treat sub-clinical mastitis will be influenced by both cow and herd factors. Herds with BMSCC in the top payment band are much less likely to treat cows with sub-clinical mastitis (elevated SCC), compared with herds which are incurring financial losses as a consequence of bulk milk payment penalties resulting from the contribution these individual high SCC cows are making to the BMSCC. However, in a herd which has identified a need to reduce the BMSCC and treatment of high SCC cows is part of the approach, careful selection of cows based on their likely response to treatment is essential. The previous mastitis history of a cow both in terms of the number of clinical cases and the number of repeat cases in the same quarter, or, for example, the number and sequence of a recent raised SCC, give an indication of duration of infection or chronicity, which has a strong influence on the chance of successful treatment. Cow selection is arguably one of the most important factors in determining the outcome of a mastitis treatment. Chronic, long-term mastitis infections have a significantly reduced chance of cure than those that are more recent.

Infusion Technique

An atraumatic clean technique is essential to avoid teat end damage or the inadvertent introduction of infection. Ideally, a 'partial infusion' technique should be used which uses a shortened tip to the intramammary syringe to limit damage to the streak canal. *See* infusion technique under treatment at drying off later in this chapter.

OBJECTIVES

Historically, objectives were to resolve clinical signs, rapidly re-permit milk sales, limit udder damage and prevent the spread of infection. However, the objectives of successful treatment have evolved as the identification of mastitic cows has become more discriminate. Cows with a slightly elevated SCC, which only a few years ago would have been deemed to be normal, are now known to be sub-clinically infected. Success is no longer to make the milk visually normal. The elimination of causal bacteria and a return of the cell count to acceptable levels are essential if the long-term aim of herd mastitis control, to consistently produce milk to the high standards required by today's marketplace, is to be achieved.

The infection status of a quarter can be evaluated in a number of ways. The change of status with or without treatment can lead to a clinical cure, resulting in the disappearance of clinical signs: a bacteriological cure resulting in an absence of the causal pathogen, a cell count cure resulting in a return to an SCC of below 200,000 cells/ml. However, some fundamental questions need to be asked: Do we need to treat? Perhaps the question should be: Why do we treat – to benefit the cow or herd in terms of health and welfare? Or to benefit the dairy farmer in terms of limiting financial loss?

The likelihood of spontaneous recovery must be weighed against the prospects of successful therapy and the additional costs incurred and benefits arising. High spontaneous clinical recovery rates in the absence of therapy and the often limited success of antibiotic treatment in effecting bacteriological cures should *not* be interpreted as a reason for abandoning the treatment of mild clinical cases. A reduction in bacterial numbers in infected quarters as a result of antibiotic treatment helps to reduce spread of infection and to improve bacteriological quality of bulk milk; both are instrumental in maintaining premium milk quality. The use of non-antibiotic preparations to treat mastitis may allow large numbers of bacteria to enter the bulk tank with a resulting bactoscan payment penalty.

What are the Chances of Success?

Increasingly, antimicrobial therapy (both milking and dry cow therapy) is matched to the pathogen profile on a farm, which tends to improve success rates; however, when assessing cure rates it is as well not to attribute all outcomes to antibiotic therapy.

It is worth remembering that:

- infections can get better despite treatment, as a consequence of self-cure
- a change of treatment resulting in a clinical improvement
  - might be due to the change
  - might have been going to happen anyway
- apparent clinical failure of treatment (clots still present)
  - may be still infected
  - may, in fact, be a bacteriological cure, but the udder damage is so severe that a clinical cure may never occur (lost quarter) or will only be evident once the udder has had sufficient time to repair. The SCC may remain elevated, despite a bacteriological cure. Antibiotics only kill bacteria, they do not heal udders.

Clinical cure rates can be up to 100 per cent but will vary according to:

- pathogen involved
- previous infection history
- duration of infection
- dose and duration of treatment.

In general, bacterial cure rates:

- are lower than clinical cure rates
- are highest for mastitis caused by Gram-negative bacteria which will
  - be relatively unaffected by antibiotic treatment
  - approach 100 per cent in mild cases
- are lower for mastitis caused by Gram-positive bacteria, apart from *Streptococcus agalactiae.*

And cure rates for *Staphylococcus aureus* or *Streptococcus uberis*

- will be significantly lower
- will be affected by antibiotic treatment
- antibiotic at drying off is more effective than during lactation
- case selection and treatment protocol can improve success rates dramatically
- realistic approach must be taken, especially with pathogens such as *Staphylococcus aureus,* where chronic (long duration) infections are common, success rates are low, and removal of the cow from the herd (culling) is often the most appropriate treatment
- culling of cows carries a 100 per cent cure rate, the infection is removed from the herd, in that cow at least, but often the infection has spread within the herd and other cows are ready to take over the mantle of the highest cell count cow in the herd.

What Drug(s) Should I Use?

This is a subject in its on right and the author would refer the reader to the further reading list for more information. Most products used to treat mastitis in dairy cows will have activity against most of the common mastitis pathogens and may contain more than one antibiotic to acheive this, giving them what is often termed broad-spectrum activity against both Gram-positive (*Staphylococci* and *Streptococci*) as well as Gram-negative bacteria such as *E. coli*. However, individual drugs within, for example, the penicillin group such as penicillin G, penethamate or cloxacillin, will have an effect only against Gram-positive bacteria. It is important to know that the product being used has at least theoretical activity against the bacteria being treated. There is little point in using penicillin to treat a known *E. coli* mastitis infection.

It is the author's opinion that cure rates (clinical, bacteriological or cell count) are more affected by factors other than the therapeutic agent used. The outcome of treatment is determined more by the case characteristics, such as causal pathogen, including strain variation, duration of infection and the duration of treatment, than by the therapeutic agent used. However, where the causal pathogen is known, experienced clinicians will often have justifiable views based on their own experiences regarding the efficacy of particular therapeutic agents against certain pathogens.

What are the Economics of Treatment?

The likelihood of spontaneous recovery must be weighed against the prospects of successful therapy, the additional costs incurred and the benefits arising. When treating a mild case of clinical mastitis with a label treatment of three tubes, the cost of the drugs used will be 20 to 30 per cent of the direct costs, whereas the cost of the discarded milk during treatment and the withhold period will be 70 to 80 per cent of the direct costs.

When deciding whether to treat sub-clinical mastitis, other factors, such as the risk of the spread of infection within the herd, the current BMSCC and any quality payment penalties currently incurred, the long-term gain of future production in the treated cow (including increased yield and age, that is the potential number of subsequent lactations) may need to be balanced against the cost of culling. At a herd level, the reduction

in individual cow SCC after treatment can have positive effect on milk value by reducing BMSCC. In certain instances, the financial calculations can be based on predictable results, such as whole-herd blitz therapy for *Streptococcus agalactiae*; but more often cure rates are more variable and cost benefits are more difficult to determine.

Pros and Cons of Treatment with Antibiotic

Pros

- increased chance of treatment success particularly with Gram-positive infections (clinical/bacteriological/SCC)
- reduced excretion of bacteria in milk and reduced spread within the herd, which impacts on BMSCC and payment penalties
- more rapid resolution of clinical signs, more rapid return of milk to bulk tank and avoidance of yield depression
- improved quality regarding fat lactose and casein
- reduced chance of recurrence of infection (either in current or subsequent lactation).

Cons

- cost of treatment (drugs) and milker's time
- cost of milk discard, which may be especially significant in high-yielding (freshly calved) cows
- risk of contamination of milk supply
- theoretical risk of increased antibiotic resistance
- aspirations to magic bullet, rather than husbandry and management to control mastitis
- may not significantly affect outcome especially in mild Gram-negative infections.

How Do I Know Whether I Have Been Successful?

Post-treatment monitoring is a valuable tool for assessing whether treatments have been successful. Lack of clinical response is relatively easy to spot as the signs of mastitis persist. However, SCC or bacteriological cure is more difficult to assess. The timing of testing will alter the result, and also to some extent its validity. Sampling too quickly after treatment has been completed may give underestimates of cure by SCC estimation and overestimates of cure with bacteriology.

SCC monitoring

- next regular monthly composite milk recording
  - advantage: cheap and paid for
  - disadvantages: composite sample; timing fixed by contract and unrelated to treatment
- ad hoc SCC (such as CMT)
  - advantages: cheap; can be performed on affected quarter; can be repeated easily and frequently
  - disadvantage: has a lower threshold of detection of 400–500,000 cells/ml unless a trace result is taken as a failure.

Bacteriology

- advantages: assesses bacteriological cure; gives identity of pathogen cultured
- disadvantages: more costly than SCC; may give false negative results, particularly soon after treatment.

An important and, in the author's opinion, underused method of assessing success is the routine post-treatment bacteriological examination of milk from treated quarters, particularly in persistent sub-clinical infections or in clinical cases where it has proved difficult to achieve a clinical cure. The timing of post-treatment sampling for bacteriological culture is important, particularly with persistent bacteria such as *Staphylococcus aureus*. There is a need to evaluate sufficiently long after the cessation of treatment. With *Streptococcus uberis*, samples can, in the author's experience, be taken for bacteriology seven to ten

days after the last treatment, although SCC may still be elevated at this point. Samples taken at twenty-one to twenty-eight days post-treatment may show more realistic bacteriological cure rates for *Staphylococcus aureus* than the artificially high, apparent bacteriological cure rates found at seven to ten days post-treatment, where suppression of infection rather than bacteriological cure may be a factor. *Staphylococcus aureus* infections can 'recover' after treatment, with excretion being suppressed for up to two to four weeks post-treatment and intermittent excretion further complicates the assessment of success rates. However, sampling at a greater time after the end of treatment does increase the chance of new infections occurring and being detected effectively increasing the failure rate.

TYPES OF 'TREATMENT' AVAILABLE

Self-cure

Self-cure is perhaps more common than is often supposed. Despite the fact that the teat orifice is continually being challenged and penetrated by bacteria, the cow's normal defence mechanisms make the establishing of infection a relatively rare occurrence. It is also possible for infections to become established and then be eliminated by self-cure at a later date. It is clear that on occasions things get better despite what we do rather than because of what we do.

Treatment during Lactation

(*See* Appendix III.) Treatment protocols, not surprisingly, have evolved with time. Historically, treatment during lactation involved the regular 'stripping out' of the infected quarter application of a variety of topical treatments and massage to encourage the 'circulation'. The advent of antimicrobials brought a magic-bullet approach and drugs were developed with varying degrees of efficacy against the common mastitis-causing pathogens. It appears that the 'normal' label three tubes used for a treatment course has become part of mastitis history, but it is difficult to find any reference to the logic by which this three-tube approach was chosen. Initially, one tube was infused and only repeated if necessary, depending on the clinical response. Gradually it became common place for 'data sheets' to suggest that three tubes were infused at intervals of 24hr (every other milking). Latterly 'data sheet treatment regimes' have tended to move towards three tubes infused every 12hr (every milking). It is felt that more 'aggressive' therapy in the early stages of infection (12 hourly tubing) gives a better chance of a bacteriological cure. This approach also benefits the producer by shortening the duration of treatment, thus reducing the amount of milk discarded during treatment and the milk withhold period. This has resulted in a bacterial infection being treated with a 'time-dependent' antibiotic, where the duration of treatment determines success rather than therapeutic drug levels, for only three treatments at intervals of 12hr for a 36hr period. Limited therapeutic dosing (short treatment courses with short withhold periods) is employed due to economic and residue-avoidance concerns. This may be contrary to what is really needed and, as a result, effective inhibitory concentrations are not maintained for periods that would normally be applied in other areas of infectious disease treatment. What would be the likely comment from a GP if a patient took 36hr of treatment of a course of antibiotic for, say, a sore throat and then complained it had not got better?

Selecting Cows for Treatment in Lactation

Clinical Mastitis Cases

It is taken as a given that all clinical cases justify treatment on welfare grounds. However, some cases may be beyond the realms of successful treatment and are regarded as being a lost quarter. Cows with lost quarters can be milked on the other three quarters provided that the acute inflammation has subsided and there is no pain nor swelling. But often the risk of contagious spread from the discharge from a severely damaged quarter will result in the cow being culled. On occasions, where cows with lost quarters are allowed to calve in again after a dry period the quarter may become productive again.

Problem Cows and Off-label Treatment

In addition to the 'normal' new clinical infection which receives treatment and is cured, there are two areas which justify special attention: persistent or repeat infected clinical and sub-clinical mastitic cows. These cows tend to have more chronic infections which do not respond well to treatment and more aggressive therapy is usually reserved for these situations where conventional treatment is known to be ineffective. These regimes are either a form of 'aggressive therapy', where more frequent treatment or increased doses are used, 'extended therapy', where treatment is prolonged in an attempt to improve success rates or 'combination therapy', where parenteral therapy (usually by injection) is combined with intramammary tubes to improve the penetration of the udder tissue and improve the success rate. Extended therapy is aimed at exposing the infection to drug levels above the MIC for longer, which, in the case of time-dependent antibiotics is closely linked with improved success rate. Aggressive therapy, increasing the dose, although not linked to improved success rate, unlike in the case of a 'concentration-dependent' antibiotic, can, in the author's opinion, improve success rates because it is getting the tissue levels above MIC that dictate killing power. So, by increasing dose rates, the diffusion into difficult areas of an inflamed mammary gland will be improved by a concentration gradient. Consequently, treatment protocols for resilient cases often involve an increase of both the dose and the duration of treatment. Extending the duration of treatment in the case of *Staphylococcus aureus* is aimed at prolonging the course beyond the life of the neutrophil and, with *Streptococcus uberis*, to overcome possible periods of bacterial dormancy. *See* relevant sections in Chapter 3.

167

- Persistently infected quarters – repeat clinical case cows – carrier cows: based ideally on the repeat isolation of the same pathogen from repeat clinical cases in the same quarter, these cows can confidently be identified as being infected with a chronic, long-term infection. Often bacteriology is not available for all samples, and assumptions have to be made. Repeat clinical cases in the same quarter and repeated isolation of the same pathogen despite treatment will help to differentiate these cows from transiently infected cows, which may have either self-cured or responded to treatment. Carrier status is most likely to be associated with *Staphylococcus aureus* or *Streptococcus uberis*. Other streptococci such as *Streptococcus dysgalactiae* or *Streptococcus agalactiae* can be relatively easily eliminated from individual infected quarters with antibiotic therapy. However, these carrier cows pose a significant infection risk to the rest of the herd and, as culling is the only alternative, they will often justify the increased expense of a specifically tailored treatment regime.
- Persistently infected quarters – sub-clinical infections – high SCC cows: persistent high SCC cows, as with repeat clinical cows, are increasingly being recognized as a significant source of infection to the uninfected cows in the herd. Research shows that many of these cows are more likely to respond to extended treatment protocols. On the other hand, for example, chronic *Staphylococcus aureus* infections may be 'untreatable' in terms of a true and lasting bacteriological cure. It is possible, however, to buy time for a dairy farmer by treating chronic *Staphylococcus aureus* infections to reduce bacterial excretion and so limit spread, while the real problem is addressed with management and husbandry changes. Many of the cows treated in this way may eventually need to be culled, but often economics dictates that not all cows which need to be culled can be done so at the beginning of an investigation. Treatment

successes are greater at drying off, but again financial pressure brought to bear by BMSCC payment penalties, may bring a sense of urgency such that it is economic to treat persistently high cell count cows in the absence of clinical signs.

In an attempt to achieve clinical, bacteriological and cell count 'cure' various treatment regimes have been employed. These types of treatment regimes are used where infections are known to be refractory to treatment and may have resulted in previous treatment failures, recurrent clinical cases or persistently elevated SCC. Any variation from the 'data sheet recommendations' will result in the voiding of the validity of the drug companies' published withhold period and is known as 'off-label' use. It is important to note that even increasing the number of tubes infused during a course of treatment will mean that individual cows will have to have either a 'standard' milk withhold period applied (currently one week), a withhold period calculated or their milk tested by a suitable 'inhibitory substance test', such as DelvoSP or ßeta s.t.a.r. before the returning of their milk to the bulk tank.

It is worth remembering that the treatment of early infection in cows selected by having a suitable history will afford better response rates than typing to treat more chronic infections with extended treatment protocols.

Treatment at Drying Off

(*See* Appendix IV.) Infusion of antibiotic into all quarters at drying off (Dry Cow Therapy) is one of the key points in the NIRD five-point mastitis control plan and has been used successfully for almost thirty years. This treatment fulfils both of the most important criteria for disease control, namely, reduction of the duration of existing infections and reduction of the new infection rate. Antibiotic therapy at drying off is more likely to be successful at eliminating intramammary infections than antibiotic therapy during lactation. For many low BMSCC herds contagious pathogens are less of a concern having eliminated *Streptococcus agalactiae* and achieved good control of *Staphylococcus aureus*. Where pathogens with an environmental component are concerned most dry cow therapy products are reasonably effective against *Streptococcus uberis* but lack activity against Gram-negative environmental bacteria, especially the coliforms. Although favoured by some farmers, there is no evidence that repeat infusions of antibiotic DCT improve cure rates, which is not surprising considering that the dispersal of product infused into a 'dry' dry udder will be poor.

Curing existing infections – advantages of dry cow therapy:

- higher cure rate, particularly for *Staphylococcus aureus*
- higher dose and longer acting antibiotic preparations can be used safely
- antibiotic is retained in the udder longer (not milked out)
- possible increased time for healing/regeneration of udder after infection is eliminated.

Preventing new infections – advantages of dry cow therapy:

- the risk of new intramammary infection is greatest during the early and the latter part of the dry period; the early part can be covered by all licensed antibiotic dry cow products, while the whole dry period (up to a hundred days) can be covered by a non-antibiotic internal teat seal.

Most antibiotic dry cow treatments provide sufficient protection after drying off so that:

- the frequency of new infections during the dry period is reduced
- the incidence of clinical mastitis in fresh calved cows may be reduced
- most have maximum activity in the first few weeks of the dry period, activity declines as the dry period progresses
- no products are able to continue to be active up to the point of calving otherwise

antibiotic residues would be a problem at the next calving.

Preventing new infections – advantages of non-antibiotic internal teat sealant:

- the frequency of new infections during the dry period is reduced
- the incidence of clinical mastitis in freshly calved cows may be reduced
- no risk of antibiotic residues, attractive for organic dairy farmers
- shown to be present for up to a hundred days.

Dry Cow Therapy Protocols

Selective Antibiotic Dry Cow Therapy

- this is where cows are identified as infected or uninfected and only infected ones receive antibiotic DCT; unfortunately, there is no rapid, cheap and accurate way of determining true infection status so uninfected cows may receive antibiotic DCT [no different from blanket DCT where all cows receive DCT], but more worrying is when infected cows may not be treated and the best chance of cure has been missed).

Antibiotic DCT or Internal Teat Seal Dry Cow Therapy

- similar concerns as with selective DCT, although all cows receive some sort of therapy, albeit the wrong one occasionally, for example, where infected cows receive only a teat seal.

Whole Herd 'Underwritten' With Internal Teat Seal and Only Infected Cows Receive Combination Teat Seal and Antibiotic DCT

- similar concerns with regard to misidentified infected cows only receiving teat seal.

All of these protocols can be improved by using an SCC threshold adjusted to increase sensitivity to reduce the chance of identifying infected cows as uninfected, for instance, 150,000 cells/ml or even 100,000 cells/ml.

Combined Antibiotic DCT and Internal Teat Seal

- many dairy herds combine the advantages of antibiotic dry cow therapy and internal teat seal, giving cure and effectively a degree of double protection in the early dry period, with the potential of prolonged protection up to the point of calving
- combination use can improve dry-period performance in both cure and protection; improved protection is obvious, but how does adding a non-antibiotic product

to cows at drying off improve dry-period cure rates? The use of internal teat seal in combination will effectively 'underwrite' many cures obtained by the antibiotic DCT by helping to prevent a new infection just before calving; before the availability of the internal teat seal several cows will have been cured by antibiotic DCT, but would be identified as a failure to cure because they were infected again just prior to calving; the author has seen combination therapy improve dry-period performance significantly.

Infusion Technique

All the benefits of dry cow therapy can be lost by poor infusion technique:

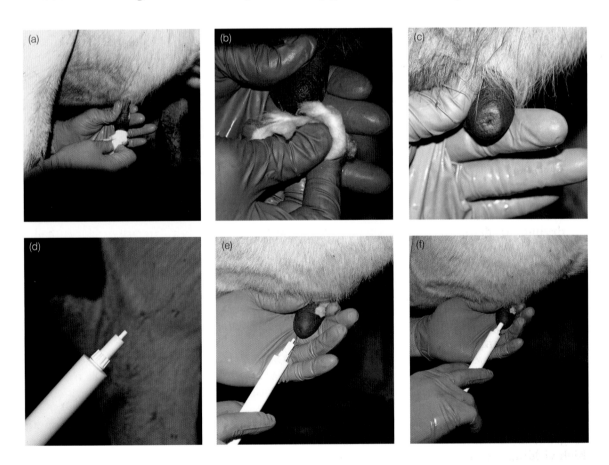

Infuse intramammary tube. (a) Swabbing teat end. (b) Swabbing teat end again. (c) Clean teat end. (d) Tube showing short tube tip. (e) Partial insertion technique. (f) Infusing product.

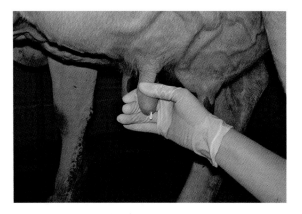

Orbeseal being stripped out of a quarter.

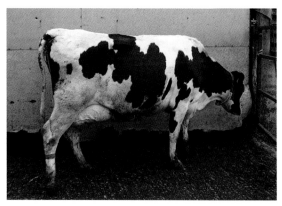

Leg tape to help to identify a treated cow.

- clean and dry each teat thoroughly (use pre-milking dip if available)
- clean the furthest pair of teats first then the nearest pair
- disinfect teat end with swabs supplied with product, or surgical- or methylated-spirit-soaked cotton wool
- infuse the dry cow tube and briefly massage each quarter, infuse the nearest pair of teats first then the furthest pair, use a partial insertion technique where possible
- dip each teat with post-milking teat dip
- keep cows penned for 30min to prevent them lying down after infusion to allow teat canal to close
- record all treatments, including cow ID, drying off date, expected calving date, product used, milk and meat withhold period, ensuring that there is sufficient time for the minimum dry period to elapse before the cow is due to calve.

Management of Cows around Drying Off

Historically, standard advice for drying off has always been to remove concentrates from the cow's ration for about one week and then abruptly stop milking. Advice is still generally that abrupt dying off is preferable to gradual. However, work has shown that high-yielding cows producing in excess of 25kg of milk per day are difficult to dry off abruptly and may be more susceptible to new intramammary infections, so once a day milking before drying off may be appropriate.

Recent research has shown an association with certain management procedures and reduced mastitis cases in the following lactation. The number of herds performing some procedures was inevitably small in some cases, but clean housing and clean infusion technique were associated with less mastitis in the following lactation, as was keeping a cow standing for 30min after infusion. However, perhaps less intuitively, a strong association with reduced mastitis in the following lactation was seen when the risk of faecal contamination in the late dry period was lessened by using a graze two weeks and rest four weeks pasture rotation, which required the heifer or dry cow paddock to be divided into three roughly equal blocks and the animals rotated every two weeks.

Drying-off Quarters

Problem cows with persistent, unresponsive clinical mastitis, high SCC and/or repeat clinical cases in one quarter may well be candidates for premature drying off of individual quarters. The quarter must be clinically normal at the time and can be dried off and left until the cow is dried off, when antibiotic dry cow is used on all four quarters. There are practical concerns, particularly on bigger farms, when more than one person milks the cows and there is a risk that the dry quarter may be inadvertently milked. When the cow recalves a proportion, often 50 to 60 per cent, will come back to production. Recent work has used 'mini dry periods', with the use of a single milking cow tube where the problem quarter is infused, not milked for seven to ten days and then the quarter is milked. The milk is discarded while the three unaffected quarters are milked and until the withhold period has elapsed and a sample from all four quarters passes an inhibitory substance test, such as DelvoSP or ßeta s.t.a.r., before returning their milk to the bulk tank.

Culling Quarters

Quarter culling where the quarter is destroyed by the use of either a single infusion of 120ml of 5 per cent Betadine (Povidine iodine solution) or of chlorhexidine infused twice with an interval of 24hr. One study of chronic *Staphylococcus aureus*-infected quarters showed that, although the treated quarter stopped milk production, *Staphylococcus aureus* could still be cultured from the Betadine-treated quarters, while the chlorhexidine appeared to return to production in the next lactation, with 50 per cent being free from *Staphylococcus aureus*. Although a single dose of NSAD (Flunixin) is used to reduce inflammation, one might assume that the procedure would be painful.

Culling

The removal of chronically infected cows is also one of the points in the NIRD five-point mastitis control plan. Culling predominantly affects the duration of infection by eliminating the cow and thus the infection from the herd. However, by removing infected cows, the new infection rate is likely to be lower because the chance of the spreading of infection is also reduced.

PRECAUTIONS WITH 'OFF-LABEL' TREATMENT

Any treatment regimen that is other than that described in the data sheet and on the label is by definition 'off-label'. All off-label treatment should be under direct veterinary supervision and should be a conscious decision for a specific situation, so appropriate precautions can be taken. In the United Kingdom 'off-label' treatment requires a minimum milk withhold of seven days and a meat withhold of twenty-eight after the last treatment. The practising veterinary surgeon has an important role to help and advise producers to ensure that no antibiotic violations occur as a result of off-label therapy. There are no recognized withhold periods for off-label treatment and it is strongly reommended that a milk sample from cows treated in this way is subjected to a recognized inhibitory substance test such as DelvoSP or ßeta s.t.a.r. before the milk is consigned to the bulk milk tank.

Types of Off-label Treatment Available

- off-label treatment types may be either:
  - intramammary
  - parentral
  - a combination of both
- there are currently only two products in the United Kingdom licensed for combination use (both using injection with a conventional, three-intramammary tube treatment)
- intramammary treatment can be:
  - aggressive (more frequent treatment or increased dosage than label recommendations)
  - extended (where treatment is for a longer period than label recommendations)
  - a combination of both
- timing of off-label treatment can be:
  - during lactation (generally at milking time)
  - during the dry period
  - treatment other than in lactation is most commonly at the start or towards the end of the dry period, since these are when the majority of antibiotics are most likely to penetrate well into

the mammary gland; they are also the most at-risk periods for new infections

- may be used in sub-clinical cases (generally identified as high SCC cows), preferably with a bacteriological sample to identify the pathogen involved; there is time to evaluate the herd situation as well as the individual cow and to choose the most appropriate treatment protocol
- may be used in clinical cases, where responses to label treatment have been shown to be poor (either failure to respond to conventional treatment or recurrence of clinical signs within a short period); ideally, once a problem is identified samples prior to the initial treatment of the next case or before a recurrent case should be taken.

ADJUNCTIVE THERAPIES

Repeat Stripping

In many infective processes the removal of infected material by a variety of means is known to be beneficial in aiding recovery. This may range from a natural defence mechanism, such as coughing up infected material in respiratory infections, to an intervention such as lancing and physically draining an abscess. Mastitis is no different, and the regular removal of infected milk from an infected quarter will aid recovery, especially in more severe cases, such as summer mastitis, where the products of infection are themselves damaging to the udder tissue.

Massaging with Topical Liniments or Embrocations

The use of the topical massage of an affected quarter is aimed at increasing the blood supply to the affected udder to encourage the natural healing process. This can be enhanced by the 'deep heat' effect that some liniments have. Their irritant nature causes the dilation of superficial capillaries and increases blood flow to the skin of the udder, much as it does when similar products are applied by athletes or other sportsmen and women to the skin of limbs with injured muscles. A word of

caution to dairy operatives: these products are irritant and can cause severe inflammation if they are inadvertently rubbed in the eye, for example, while wiping sweat away from the face in hot weather. Repeat stripping and massaging is often called 'rub and strip' and is a well accepted way of encouraging the draining of an infected mammary gland by stimulating blood circulation and possibly oxytocin release, combined with the removal of infected material from the gland.

Oxytocin

Oxytocin is frequently used to aid the stripping of infected quarters. In a very severely inflamed gland there may be pain associated with the alveoli and ducts becoming blocked with mastitis milk, which could be exacerbated by the constricting effects of oxytocin on the myoepithelial cells. However, research using high doses (100iu) of oxytocin have been shown to open the 'tight cell junctions' between the secretory cells in the udder, allowing inflammatory products to leak from the blood into the lumen of the gland, where the bacteria are likely to be, which can be beneficial. This should be under veterinary supervision and not used in pregnant cows.

Oral or Intravenous Fluid

The more severe (per-acute) forms of mastitis can result in cows being very sick and developing toxic shock, which is not infrequently accompanied by diarrhoea. As a result, the circulation is impaired and the animal often progresses to become significantly dehydrated. Corrective fluid therapy will help restore circulation as well as reduce the dehydration. Cows are clearly large animals and the volumes required are considerable.

Oral fluids are generally best delivered by stomach tube since the volumes required, often 20ltr or more, preclude drenching as a viable alternative to deliver sufficient. Stirrup pumps have been used for many years to speed the delivery of the volumes required and generally a gag is used to prevent the cow from chewing the tube. More recently, a system with an integral,

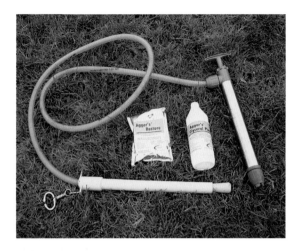

Stomach tube with integral gag and pump with products commonly used.

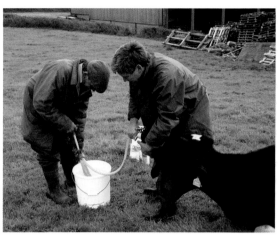

Delivering fluids by stomach tube.

robust tube with a metal spiral within the wall to stiffen it, gag and pump has become commonplace in the United Kingdom. This system means that many more cattle now receive fluid therapy because it is easily performed by a single operator, if the cow is restrained. Alternatives, with the use of a watering can or drenching with a bottle, are far less effective.

Intravenous fluids can also be used and there is a choice of using high volumes of isotonic fluid (where the concentration is much as in normal blood) or hypertonic (where the concentration is greater than that in blood). The volumes required for isotonic fluid are often in excess of 20ltr and it is advisable to avoid an excess of potassium, which can occur with lactated Ringer's solution or Hartman's solution. Often human 5ltr peritoneal lavage bags can be used (0.9 per cent normal saline Travenol). Various pressurized delivery systems have been devised, and the use of flexible 'airline' hosing can help to prevent the complications of twisted and kinked giving sets (delivery pipes). Unsurprisingly, the volumes when hypertonic saline is used are much less and are often of only 2 or 3ltr. The lower volume of fluid delivered when using hypertonic saline is hoped to be augmented by the cow immediately drinking significant quantities of water. In the author's experience, this response is variable,

with some cows drinking faster than a mains supply of water into a bucket to, on occasions, no water being drunk at all. If insufficient water is drunk after administering hypertonic saline intravenously from 10 to 20ltr of water should be administered immediately by stomach tube or pump.

Anti-inflammatory Drugs

Corticosteroids

Corticosteroids may be useful in the early stages of an inflammatory process but are of little value when dealing with established infections. Their effects are many and varied, including anti-inflammatory properties, but they also have a potentially negative impact on the immune system (immunosuppression), particularly with prolonged use, which can be counterproductive in infectious conditions such as mastitis. They have virtually no analgesic properties and so have been effectively superseded by NSAIDs.

Some intramammary antibiotic preparations contain corticosteroids, but there is some debate as to how much this is to reduce any irritant effects of the antibiotic and how much is to do with eliciting a significant anti-inflammatory effect within the udder. When used by injection, the stage of pregnancy needs to be established as they cause premature birth (abortion) in cows, particularly in their last third of pregnancy (trimester).

Non-steroidal Anti-inflammatory Drugs (NSAIDs)

NSAIDs possess several properties which make them useful for treating severe cases of mastitis in particular. As their name suggests, they are non-steroidal and are non-narcotic analgesics with potent anti-inflammatory (reduce inflammation), anti-endotoxic (help to protect the cow against endotoxic shock) and anti-pyretic (reduce the cow's increased temperature) effects. The fact that they are non-steroidal means they do not have many of the potentially negative effects of corticosteroids and, as non-narcotic pain relievers, they do not have the milk withhold issues that narcotic pain-relieving drugs would have. In fact, no narcotic drugs are licensed for dairy cows. All of these properties are beneficial to the mastitic cow. In very sick animals their use will help to make the cow feel better by reducing its high temperature, get it to recover its appetite more quickly and may help to reduce udder swelling. There is an increasing awareness that mastitis is a painful condition and that, despite the fact that NSAIDs tend be used for their anti-inflammatory properties, their analgesic qualities are often underestimated.

Calcium

It is thought that some cows with toxic mastitis are hypocalcaemic (low blood calcium), as is seen in milk fever. It is difficult to determine the cause or association. Milk fever is a risk factor for developing a toxic mastitis, but may be more due to an increased chance of recumbency and physiological changes to the cow, rather than a direct effect on the udder. However, many clinicians will give intravenous calcium to toxic mastitis cases, perhaps more as a precautionary treatment to avoid further complications of milk fever and recumbency in an already sick cow.

ALTERNATIVE THERAPIES

Various other alternative therapies are used in treating cows with mastitis, but many are unproven. Some treatments, such as cold hosing, may help to reduce inflammation, as opposed to massaging with topical liniments and embrocations already referred to, such as Uddermint or aloe vera, which results in a deep-heat effect and may help by increasing circulation.

Other treatments which make claims to have a therapeutic effect should by law be tested to show safety, efficacy and be assessed for their environmental impact, just like any other medicinal product, and, as they are being used on food-producing animals, they should have a published milk (and meat) withhold time. This would particularly apply to unlicensed products which are infused into the udder of cows for the treatment of mastitis and would include intramammary products containing aloe vera and tea tree oil.

CHAPTER EIGHT

Summer Mastitis

Summer mastitis is almost like a separate disease when the epidemiology (the way it 'works') is compared that to other types. Summer mastitis is neither contagious nor environmental in origin, but its spread is linked to the sheep headfly *Hydrotaea irritans*. Clinical disease most often occurs in non-lactating dairy cattle (dry cows) at pasture during the summer months, giving rise to the common name of 'August bag'. Summer mastitis also occurs in beef cows and is occasionally seen in calves and even bulls. It is not uncommon in northern European countries, including the United Kingdom, Denmark, Holland and Germany, often being associated with sandy, well-drained soil which is suitable for foraging, soil-dwelling insect larvae. The disease is often seen on low lying, sheltered pasture near a water course, such as a stream with nearby woodland and often with a significant number of thistles or weeds.

CAUSE

A number of bacteria have been associated with summer mastitis infection, with the most common being *Arcanobacterium pyogenes* (formerly *Corynebacterium* then *Actinomyces pyogenes*) and *Streptococcus dysgalactiae*, although the severity seems to be moderated by the presence of a variety of anaerobic bacteria, with *Peptococcus indolicus* being the most common, but *Bacteroides melaninogenicus* and *Fusobacterium necrophorum* may also be

present. It is not entirely clear how these bacteria gain entry to the udder, although via the streak canal would seem likely in the light of successful experimental inoculation through the streak canal or the frequency that summer mastitis will follow teat damage.

How Do the Bacteria Invade the Udder?

Arcanobacterium pyogenes and *Peptococcus indolicus* are ubiquitous in the bovine environment, with *Arcanobacterium pyogenes* commonly being isolated from abscesses in cattle.

- *External* (exogenous): bacterial contamination of the teat skin or orifice, particularly with infected skin lesion followed by invasion through the teat duct
- *Internal* (endogenous): bacteria enter the gland from other parts of the body, either draining via the supramammary lymph node from other infected lesions, or haematogenous spread (via blood) from other sites.

In reality, there will be a mixture of routes.

Despite the link to the sheep headfly *Hydrotaea irritans*, experimental transmission by this route has so far failed. Primary invasion of the mammary gland appears to be by either the anaerobic organism *Peptococcus indolicus* or *Streptococcus dysgalactiae*, which is then followed by *Arcanobacterium pyogenes* infection. The link to *Hydrotaea irritans* is supported by much circumstantial evidence, such as the fact that it is the most frequent visitor to the teats of cattle and peak incidence of disease occurs when the flies are most frequent on cattle. *Hydrotaea irritans* commonly carries mixtures of summer mastitis-causing bacteria. Infections more commonly occur in front quarters, which flies can reach more easily without being swished off by the animal's tail, and the control of flies in general reduces the incidence of summer mastitis.

Fly spread is clearly important, particularly in the high incidence period in the summer. However, other means of spread must occur because sporadic cases can occur at any time of the year, even in the winter. These cases may come from an infected teat lesion, heavily contaminated teat or endogenous spread from another infected focus.

Once a case has occurred, further cases may appear in the herd by mechanical transfer via inanimate fomite spread, such as discharges on bedding or via bodily contact, or animate fomite spread by flies from infected animals to other quarters, either in the same cow or between cows. Bacteria can remain viable in the gut of flies for several days and be present at subsequent feeding bouts.

The number of cases will vary from sporadic to an explosion of cases, and particularly in bad fly seasons where no fly control is attempted. The number of cases will also be governed by the number and density of animals at risk (dry cows), with more occurring when there are more animals at risk. Ensuring good husbandry as well as fly control, including an adequate level and quality of nutrition to avoid stress, will all help to maximize the cow's immune defences.

CLINICAL SIGNS

The early signs of summer mastitis are characteristic and often observant farmers can pick up the disease early and differentiate it from other mastitis. These typical early signs are a swollen teat of the affected quarter(s), showing an increase in both length and diameter sometimes a week or more before the heifer or cow becomes ill. Other early signs include flies clustering around the affected teat orifice, attracted by the secretions from the teat; these cause considerable irritation, resulting in frequent kicking. As the disease progresses, the inflamed quarter becomes hard, swollen and painful, producing a thick yellow secretion with a typical unpleasant smell. Unless recognized and treated early in the disease's progression, the infection advances to the point where it effectively becomes an abscess in the quarter. As a result of this often necrotizing infection, the associated poisons cause massive, often irreversible damage to the udder, resulting in a lost quarter. These poisons (toxins) are absorbed into the blood stream, causing a toxaemia and making the animal initially lethargic, but often progressing to oedema (swelling) of the hind legs, resulting in lameness, separation from the group, lack of appetite and loss in body condition. If left untreated, and sometimes even with treatment, the systemic effects of summer mastitis can result in abortions and even the death of the affected animal. As a consequence of in-calf, non-lactating (dry) cattle not being milked twice a day, the observation of them can be sporadic and so summer

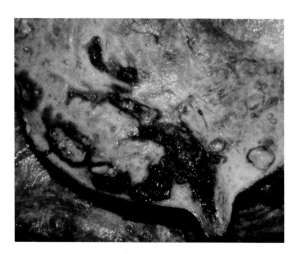

Cross-section of a quarter affected by summer mastitis; note the multiple abscessation.

mastitis, once discovered, may well be quite advanced.

Some fresh calved cows appear to be affected with a pure *Arcanobacter pyogenes* infection which is less severe than full-blown summer mastitis, but is nonetheless difficult to treat. The author has found a combination treatment of Mamayzin (Boehringer Ingelheim Ltd) and extended treatment with tubes to improve success rates. A post-treatment bacteriology sample is advisable.

TREATMENT

Although the bacteria involved are Gram-positive and highly sensitive to penicillin, some reports, including the author's experience, suggest oxytetracycline to be more effective. It is very rare to 'save' the quarter, and secretory function after calving is unlikely in the affected quarter. Parentral administration (injection) of oxytetracycline is used to keep the animal healthy, combined with repeated stripping out of the infected quarter to drain what is effectively a glorified abscess. Infusion of antibiotic tubes in the evening is sensible, unless the farmer is going to stay up all night stripping the quarter! Frequency of stripping is dictated by how much pus is removed. In the early stages stripping every two to three hours can be very helpful in avoiding the effects of toxaemia, especially if reasonable quantities can be removed by stripping. However, if as little as a few millilitres are stripped out, as is often the case in very hard swollen udders, then the interval can be extended. Despite antibiotic therapy and regular stripping of the affected quarter(s), the affected glands are highly unlikely to be functional and often become hard and indurated. Occasionally, pus may drain through the skin from a superficial abscess in the affected gland. Once diagnosed, it is critical that the animal is removed from the group at the first opportunity to reduce the chance of spread. The hopeless treatment response in summer mastitis emphasizes the need for effective preventive measures.

CONTROL

Deciding which control methods are the most useful is difficult for vet, farmer and research worker alike. There appear to be good and bad years for summer mastitis, such that some research workers have been frustrated in their trial work by getting no cases in their control group (no preventive control methods group), which makes assessing the benefits of the several control methods difficult, to say the least. However, there are some control methods that most would agree are useful.

The control of summer mastitis is based mainly on fly control and the use of antibiotic dry cow preparation. Repeating dry cow preparations after three weeks in very high risk situations has been advocated by some workers. Internal teat seal has also been used, either alone or in combination with antibiotic dry cow preparations.

- dry cow treatment on all cows
  - antibiotic DCT
  - repeat in three weeks in very high risk herds
  - possible use of internal teat seal
  - in herds with high in-calf heifer summer mastitis rates, heifers can be treated but it can be dangerous for both heifer and operator; use a non-insertion technique to avoid damaging the streak canal
- fly control from before fly activity begins, for instance, June–October; pour-ons or fly tags
  - ear tags give good protection against flies for the head, but less so for the abdomen and udder
  - there was a fashion to use two ear tags simultaneously
  - pour-on/spot-on can be applied direct to the udder as well as the back (the author favours 25 per cent of dose being applied direct to the udder, with a small spot on the forehead and the rest on the back)

- limit fly attack
  - maintain good teat condition to limit fly attack – abrasive plants such as thistles can result in abrasions on teats
  - possible use of teat bandages, for instance, Leukopor tape and Leuko spray aerosol, barriers such as Stockholm tar or repellents applied to teats
- pasture management
  - avoid high risk pastures
    - low lying pasture near water courses (streams/rivers)
    - wooded areas adjoining fields
  - pasture on hilltop is likely to keep wind speed >20km/hr which will discourage flies from venturing out from woodland and bushes to feed on cattle
- maintain good dry cow nutrition
- possible housing of dry cows: *Hydrotaea irritans* tends not to enter buildings
- in extreme situations a change to the calving pattern to reduce/avoid animals at risk
  - may be only alternative in organic herds at mastitis risk in high summer.
- monitor animals: close inspection at least twice daily, segregate any suspect animals immediately to limit spread.

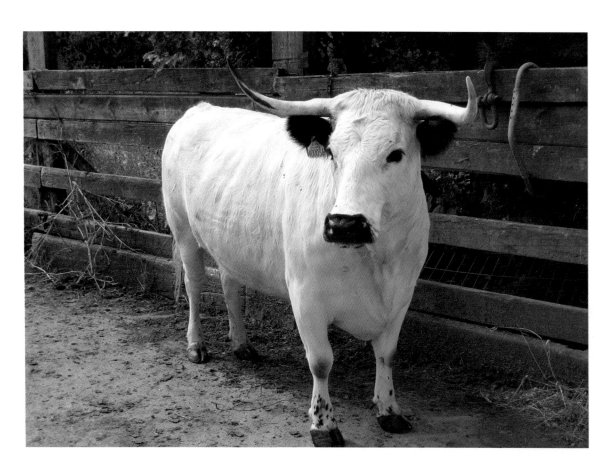

White Park cow.

CHAPTER NINE

Udder and Teat Conditions Predisposing to Mastitis

Conditions affecting the udder and or teats, while not being mastitis themselves, can and often do predispose cows to mastitis. Some may be variations of normal physiological changes, such as excessive udder oedema or abnormalities such as blood in the milk or a 'pea' in the teat, while others may have a physical or infectious cause.

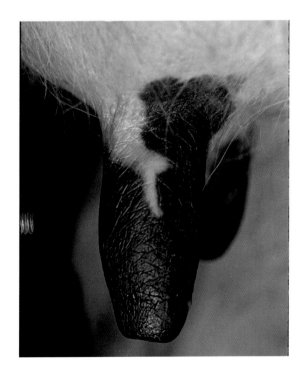

Normal teat.

NON-INFECTIOUS UDDER AND TEAT SKIN CONDITIONS

There are a number of conditions affecting the skin of the udder and teat which can have a significant impact on the risk of a cow developing mastitis.

Generalized Skin Conditions

Sunburn seen in non-pigmented (white) udder and skin, will be restricted to areas exposed to direct sunlight and so may affect only one side of a teat.

Photosensitization reaction within the skin between photoreactive chemicals (most commonly St John's wort in the United Kingdom) and sunlight. The reaction is to light rather than direct sunlight and so will not be restricted to areas of skin exposed to direct sunlight. However, the reaction is affected by the degree of exposure, and so more exposed areas, especially pale or white ones, will be more severely affected. The skin initially becomes thickened and painful, goes like cardboard and then sloughs or peels off. Some cows will recover while others seem to be permanently affected, with the condition being less severe in winter. Reports of liver function abnormalities resulting in photosensitization might explain some of these non-transient cases.

Wet eczema most commonly seen in heifers in the groin between the udder and the hind leg and can be likened to nappy (diaper) rash. Treatments are numerous and varied, including washing in salt water, udder creams and drying antibiotic sprays. As is often the case, improving a skin condition is a balance between drying out to reduce the chance of bacterial growth and moisturizing the skin to aid healing. Wet eczema can become so severe

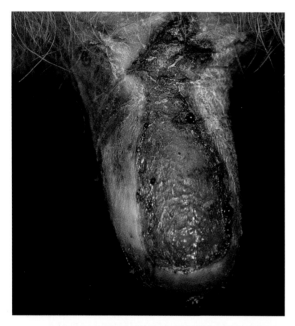

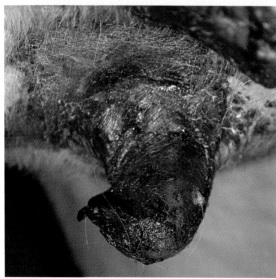

Two cases of teat necrosis.

that the animal is impossible to milk and, on rare occasions, may even result in its being culled.

Teat necrosis, seen in heifers, has been recognized in recent years in many countries, including the United Kingdom There seems to be an association with over-fat and possibly older heifers, or at least excessive oedema may be playing a part. There may be a nutritional component in terms of protein and fluid leakage or accumulation. The skin of the teat goes hard like cardboard and often has a purple colour. The affected skin can slough and the whole teat become hard. It appears to be a disturbance to the normal blood supply and/or drainage to the teat, such that, as a result of, one assumes, pain or discomfort, self-mutilation can result in the teats' being licked severely, making them even more sore and in extreme cases actually bitten off.

Udder Oedema

A degree of oedema in cows around calving is unavoidable as the cow readies herself for the huge alteration in vascular flow occurring during the change from a dry to a lactating gland. However, it is not uncommon, particularly in heifers, to see this become excessive to the point that 'pitting oedema' is detectable.

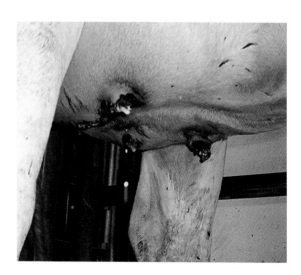

Heifer self-traumatized and licked/chewed teats off.

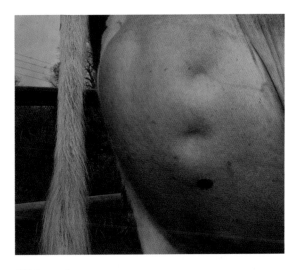

Udder oedema.

This condition occurs when a 'pit' can be left after applying pressure with a finger to the surface of, in this case, the udder.

Consequences

- painful – making milking difficult
- predisposes to mastitis
- severe cases result in loss of viability of skin, leading to sloughing
- in extreme cases can lead to culling.

Control

- may be a heritable component?
- diet
- avoid overfeeding ('steaming up') prior to calving
- avoid excess protein and or salts (minerals) intake pre-calving
- ensure adequate exercise pre-calving – limb movement improves fluid drainage through the lymphatic system, avoiding increased fluid retention.

Blood in Milk

Blood in milk can vary from a few blood clots, to milk that essentially looks like blood in all four quarters. While milk is visibly abnormal it will have to be discarded, resulting in financial loss to the farmer. Although quite dramatic, often the long-term consequences are not as significant as one might suppose. Work has shown that, although milk with obvious blood content has a raised SCC initially when compared to milk from quarters without a visible blood content, this had disappeared by seven to fourteen days after calving. Cows producing milk with obvious blood content are no more likely to yield a bacteriological growth when sampled at calving, and there is no difference in the mastitis rate in the first 100 days after calving. There are no recognized effective treatments, although milking just enough to check for mastitis and flush bacteria from the udder may help by increasing back pressure within the udder, simulating the applying of pressure to a cut to stem blood flow.

INFECTIOUS UDDER AND TEAT SKIN CONDITIONS

Most teat skin conditions can be treated by using the usual post-milking teat-conditioning teat dips (containing emollients and humectants), which will be active against both mastitis-causing bacteria and viruses.

Bovine Herpes Mamillitis (BHM)

BHM is a viral condition seen sporadically in the United Kingdom, with perhaps the most common occurrence in the autumn/winter. Dairy cows are more frequently affected, although it also can be seen in beef cows. The condition is more severe in heifers as they are less likely to have immunity, sometimes resulting in significant spread. The source of infection is not always clear, but, in common with other herpes viruses, stress such as calving can reactivate carrier cows. The reaction to infection can vary from undetectable (apart from production of antibodies conferring immunity), through mild lesions which heal rapidly, to severely painful erosive lesions. In the acute phase vesicles containing huge numbers of virus particles burst and release a highly infectious fluid, which can be spread by milking machine, milkers' hands and flies.

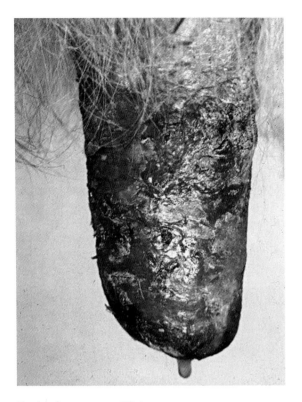

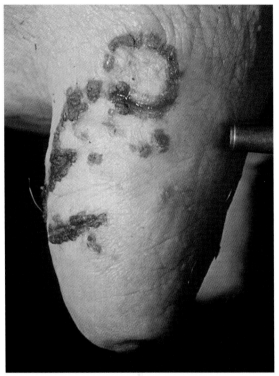

Bovine herpes mamillitis.

Pseudocowpox.

Affected animals should ideally be milked last or the milking unit disinfected. Recovered animals develop immunity and recurrence in the same animal is rare.

Pseudocowpox

This is a viral condition generally more common but much less severe than BHM, resulting in classic horseshoe-shaped lesions. It is caused by a parapox virus which is closely related to sheep orf virus, thus increasing the chance of seeing this condition in herds with close contact with sheep. There does not appear to be a seasonal variation in cases, and, as immunity is poor, there may be recurrence. Early stages show a reddening of the teat skin, which progresses to pustules which rupture and form scabs which heal outwards after ten to twelve days, resulting in a characteristic ring or horseshoe-shaped scab.

The virus can also affect human skin, sometimes resulting in 'milker's nodule', which will also tend to scab and heal. Repeat cycling of infection can occur within the herd as well as between milker and herd; this may be limited by the wearing of gloves while milking. Pseudocowpox should not be confused with cowpox, last seen in a cow in the United Kingdom in 1978, which is caused by a virus closely related to the vaccinia virus and used by Edward Jenner in 1796 for the immunization of patients against variola virus (smallpox). This was the first known vaccination of a human patient, which eventually contributed to the effective eradication of smallpox from the world and gave us the name vaccination.

Bovine Papillomatosis (Teat Warts)

Bovine papilloma viruses cause papillomatosis or warts on teats, with purportedly up to six strains of papilloma virus of which at least two are identified as the cause of warts on teats. Warts are most common on young cows and there is considerable variation in their appearance. Filamentous warts, often with frond-like protuberances of up to 2cm, are the most problematical in terms of mastitis risk, and, on occasions, newly calved heifers may have their teats completely obscured by them. The mastitis risks increase if the warts are near the teat orifice since they can interfere with both hygiene and milk flow. They may also increase mastitis risk by interfering with the airtight liner attachment, causing liner slips or by making the cow kick the clusters off since they are sensitive to touch.

Warts are easily damaged and bleed, occasionally profusely and particularly if they are 'plucked' off the teat to remove them.

Autogenous vaccines (made from harvested wart material) have been used to try to boost immunity to encourage shedding of the warts in severe cases where a batch of heifers are affected. These vaccines are unlicensed, not always successful and can strictly be used only on the animal from which the warts were harvested. Many frond warts will, however, resolve over the first lactation, although some are persistent and may need to be removed surgically. Other types of wart are also common, with white, smooth, flat ones occurring anywhere on the teat surface, often without causing any problem in milking or mastitis.

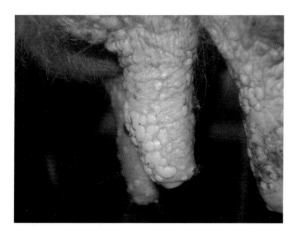

Flat warts on teat.

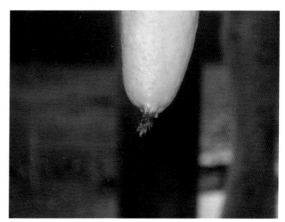

Wart on the end of a teat which looks similar to hyperkeratosis.

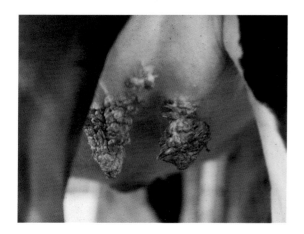

Extensive, filamentous warts on all four teats.

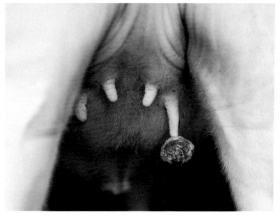

Large wart on teat end.

Other Infectious Causes of Teat Lesions

Foot-and-mouth (FMD) and bluetongue (BT) can both give rise to severe teat lesions.

PHYSICAL INJURIES TO THE TEAT AND UDDER

Physical injuries will include those caused by mechanical trauma from cuts, treads and crushed teats, as well as milking machine-induced hyperkeratosis of the teat end, to environmental damage such as may be caused by chemicals from, for example, incorrectly diluted teat dip chemical or from exposure-type damage to wet, cold and windy weather.

Blackspot

Although primarily an infection of the teat orifice, most often with *Fusiformis necrophorum*, there is invariably a degree of milking machine-induced teat-end damage. The infection erodes the teat orifice, which may become occluded, leading to incomplete and very slow milking. Often the milker will have to scratch the teat end to make milking possible, which causes additional damage to the teat orifice increasing further the risk of mastitis by other mastitis-causing bacteria. On occasions, a teat cannula is inserted to facilitate milk removal, but even this can increase the risk of mastitis. Blackspot, in the author's experience, seems recently to have become less common. The complete cessation of milking of the affected quarter for from seven to ten days has been found to be successful in aiding healing. A couple of squirts of milk may be removed by hand to check for mastitis and remove bacteria, but the teat end is given a chance to heal by not being subjected to trauma from the milking machine twice a day.

Cut Teats

Although some minor teat cuts can be successfully repaired by using tape, with or without aerosol spray glue, if the cuts are penetrating the milk canal suturing is the preferred method

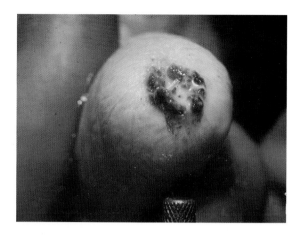

Blackspot.

of repair, although staples can be used but will require veterinary intervention. To consider the wide variety of types of cut teat individually is beyond the scope of this book. On occasions, particularly with fistulae penetrating the teat lumen, surgical repair can be delayed until the cow is dry as surgical wound healing is improved by the animal's not being exposed to the traumas of twice-a-day milking.

Crushed Teats

The individual approach will depend on the severity of the injury, but as with blackspot, to cease milking for from one to two weeks will give the best results.

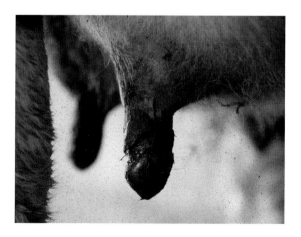

Cut teat.

185

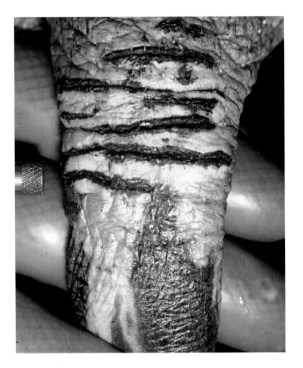

Chapped teat.

Chapped Teats

Chaps are effectively cracks in the skin which break its waterproofing and allow bacterial colonization. Chaps are most common in cold, wet and dirty conditions and will be exacerbated by wind chill. Post-milking disinfection (ideally by dipping) with products containing high proportions of emollients and humectants, such as glycerine or lanolin, will help the conditioning of the teat and aid healing.

Other Machine-induced Changes and Damage to Teats

Some changes seen in teat shape or damage can be directly attributed to the effects of a milking machine. These include those that are likely to be rapidly reversible, such as teat- end oedema, congestion, ringing, wedging and teat discoloration, as well as more durable changes, such as teat-end haemorrhage, either as small petechia or larger areas, and perhaps the most important change influencing mastitis rates, hyperkeratosis of the teat orifice.

Hyperkeratosis of the Teat Orifice

The keratin lining of the streak canal is sticky and is part of the udder defence mechanism trapping bacteria. Particularly during machine milking, some keratin is extruded from the streak canal; this is described as hyperkeratosis. Abnormal milking-machine function, such as excess vacuum or an inadequate pulsation massage phase, will exacerbate this extrusion. Hyperkeratosis describes the teat end through a range of changes from a thickened smooth keratin ring, to extending fronds of keratin around the teat orifice. Despite what one might

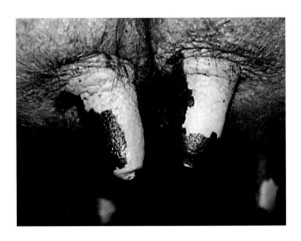

Overmilking resulting in the visible ringing of teats.

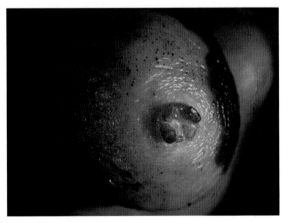

Petichae on teat end.

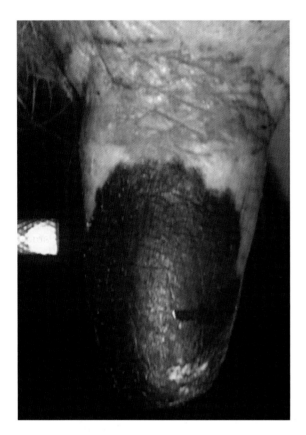

Bruised teat from mouthpiece trauma.

longer unit-on times with machine-milked cows. When scores for all teat ends are used little or no correlation has been shown between teat-orifice hyperkeratosis and intramammary infection. However, when the individual classification of teat ends was considered, those teats with a greater than mild or moderate degree of hyperkeratosis and roughness did have an increased probability of new infection. The damage to the teat end allows colonization by mastitis-causing bacteria, while simultaneously reducing the streak canal defence mechanism. Increased colonization, in association with a high hyperkeratosis score, may increase the risk of mastitis and will be more significant in the absence of post-milking disinfectant.

Hyperkeratosis Scoring

An international group of mastitis workers, known as the Teat Club International (TCI), has developed a teat-scoring system that is both reliable and simple. Using a four-point teat-end scoring method, with one normal score (N) and three abnormal scores (S, R and VR), herds can be assessed for this condition of perhaps the most important area of a dairy cow. Poor teat-end condition, particularly at the higher scores, is associated with an increased risk of mastitis.

expect, hyperkeratosis has been observed in hand-milked and beef cows, but, unsurprisingly, is commonly observed in dairy cows. Research suggests that the degree of hyperkeratosis increases as milk yield increases or with

Observation of Teat Condition Immediately after Milking as a Tool

The effects of the milking machine on the teat can be assessed immediately after

Teat Club International hyperkeratosis score

N	Normal	No ring, the teat end is smooth with a small even orifice.
S	Mild	Smooth or slightly rough ring with a raised ring around the orifice. The raised area may be smooth or slightly rough. No keratin fronds are present.
R	Moderate	Rough ring with raised, roughened ring with fronds of keratin extending 1–3 mm from the orifice.
VR	Severe	Very rough ring with keratin extending more than 4 mm from the orifice. The rim of the ring may often be cracked.

milking by observing teat congestion, shape and colour, including haemorrhages, as well as hyperkeratosis. The use of a head torch will aid observation particularly of the teat end. Observation of cow comfort levels during milking, using indicators such as fidgeting or kicking at the milking unit, and particularly at low flow periods at the end of milking, will also give an indication of teat congestion.

Observation of the whole herd is ideal, but this can be too time-consuming and disruptive to the milking routine. Often a random selection of eighty cows or 20 per cent of the herd, whichever is greater, will give a useful indication of teat-end condition within the herd. If more than 20 per cent of teat scores are R or VR, or more than 10 per cent are VR then both the milking routine and the milking machine warrant further investigation.

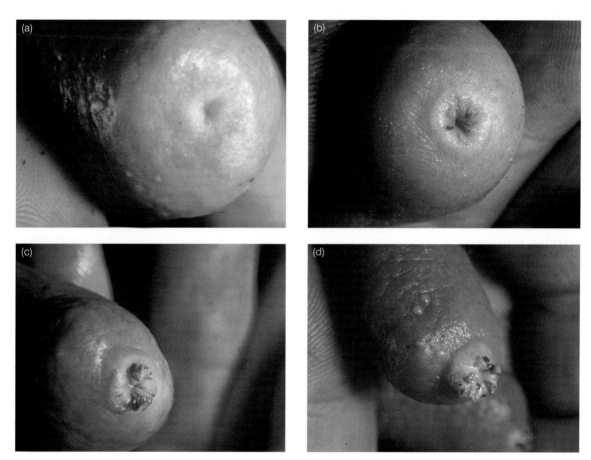

Hyperkeratosis. (a) Score N (normal). (b) Score S (mild – smooth). (c) Score R (moderate – rough). (d) Score VR (severe – very rough).

APPENDIX I

Minimizing Mastitis in Your Herd

Minimizing mastitis involves following a recognized mastitis control plan to lower new infection rates and the duration of infection by the application of appropriate management techniques and therapy in both lactation and the dry period. However, unless the introduction of specific mastitis pathogens on to the farm is also avoided, by either avoiding the introduction of infected cattle or by the potential introduction by shared farm staff, many of the benefits of good mastitis management will be lost.

Are you mastitis disease-risk averse or mastitis disease-risk tolerant?

Biosecurity for mastitis is simpler than for many other infectious diseases. The risks of the incursion of mastitis pathogens on to a farm are largely based around the introduction of cattle carrying pathogens, with mastitis pathogens forming the greatest risk. However, there are risks with personnel, and relief milkers pose a risk of introducing *Staphylococcus aureus*, particularly if they do not wear gloves for milking. Environmental pathogens, as their name implies, are present if not ubiquitous in the farm environment and their introduction on to a farm is not relevant.

BIOSECURITY LEVELS (1 = LOW RISK, 5 = HIGH RISK)

1. Closed herd – no cattle enter farm – all home-bred by artificial insemination (AI), embryo transfer (ET) or natural service by home-bred bull
2. No entry of new cattle, but return of existing cattle allowed (for instance, show cattle)
3. Entry of new cattle (known medical records and appropriate pre- and post-purchase tests) with isolation and/or quarantine

4. Entry of new cattle (known medical records) with no or incomplete isolation or quarantine
5. Entry of new cattle (no medical records) and no isolation.

Steps in Formulating a Farm-specific Biosecurity Plan

1. Identify risk pathways for incursion on to farm of specific mastitis pathogens
2. Assess the risk that such pathogens will be introduced
3. Assess the risk that, if the specific mastitis pathogens were introduced, how rapidly they would spread
4. Target your programme to address the highest risk activities or loop-holes in your system.

The major risks for mastitis pathogen incursion onto a dairy farm are *Streptococcus agalactiae*, *Staphylococcus aureus*, and possibly *Mycoplasma bovis*, although the latter is currently a rare pathogen of the udder in the United Kingdom.

If cattle have to be brought on to a dairy farm, that is, maintaining a closed herd will not be possible, then purchasing from known status herds, coupled with individual cow testing is advisable.

Many herds purchasing cattle will rely on the BMSCC of the source herd, or possibly the individual SCC of the cows to be purchased. It is rare for milk from purchased cattle to be bacteriologically cultured. The author has had several experiences of both *Streptococcus agalactiae* and *Staphylococcus aureus* brought into apparently free herds via purchased cattle, with significant financial consequences, as well as one case where a relief milker appeared to introduce *Staphylococcus aureus* on to a farm.

Checklist for Investigation

CLINICAL MASTITIS RECORDS

- Incidence: number of cases per 100 cows per year
- Severity: sick cows or even fatalities
- Response to treatment: recurrence rates
- Stage of lactation: fresh calved or later in lactation
- Seasonality: time of year
- Age of cows affected: heifers or older cows

SUB-CLINICAL MASTITIS RECORDS SCC

- BMSCC
- Individual SCC records
  - new infection rates
  - non-recovered new infection rates
  - dry-period performance

COWS

- Clinical mastitis detection and treatment protocols
- Teat score: 20 per cent of herd or 80 cows, whichever is greater
- Cleanliness: hygiene score
- Condition scoring: changes in body condition
- Faecal scoring: nutrition
- Other health concerns: such as, milk fever and displaced abomasums BVD etc

MILKING PROCESS

- Vacuum level
- Pulsation rate and ratio
- Liner slips
- Liner replacement interval
- Teat preparation, including pre-dip

- Teat drying
- Foremilk checking
- Lag time
- Overmilking
- Slow milking
- Cluster removal (ACRs)
- Post-milking teat disinfection
- Washing water tank
- Cluster disinfection

HOUSING CUBICLES

- Bedding: sand, straw, sawdust, recycled paper
- Base: e.g. mattress, mat
- Size: length, width
- Head rail/brisket board: position
- Dung channel: number of times a day scraped out
- Overcrowding: stocking rate
- General hygiene: overall cleanliness
- Humidity/ventilation

HOUSING YARDS

- Bedding: sand, straw, sawdust, recycled paper
- Water trough position: wet bedding
- Access points in and out of bedded area
- Overcrowding: stocking rate
- General hygiene: overall cleanliness
- Humidity/ventilation

OTHER AVAILABLE DATA

- BMSCC
- Bacteriology results
- Bactoscan
- Milk-machine test report

APPENDIX III: Herd Protocol for the Approach to Treatment in Lactation

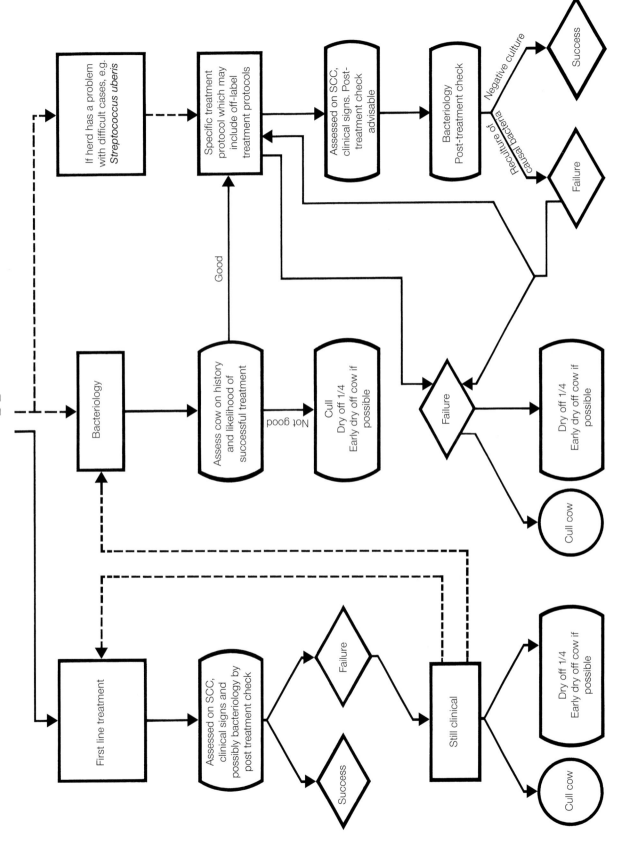

APPENDIX IV

Flowchart for Approach to Drying Off

See diagram overleaf.

1 ALL COWS NO TREATMENT

This was clearly the approach before the availability of any treatment at drying off; tends to be used by only a few organic herds.

- *Pros*: no products introduced into the udder.
- *Cons*: misses an opportunity for cure and protection from new infections.

2 ALL COWS ANTIBIOTIC DCT

Historically this was the first improved approach to cows at drying off.

- *Pros*: aimed at cure and gives some protection against early dry-period infection.
- *Cons*: does not protect in late dry period.

3 MOST COWS ANTIBIOTIC DCT, WITH SOME SELECTED LOW SCC COWS ORBESEAL ONLY

Early use of Orbeseal, an internal teat seal (Pfizer Animal Health) in the United Kingdom.

Alternate use of either antibiotic DCT or Orbeseal.

Later became 4 (see below).

- *Pros*: uninfected cows, if correctly identified, protected.
- *Cons*: poor tools available to detect infected or uninfected cows, so:
  - uninfected cows might receive antibiotic DCT, no change to 2.
  - infected cows wrongly identified as uninfected and best chance of cure in dry period missed.

4 ALL COWS ORBESEAL AND SELECTED COWS ANTIBIOTIC DCT

Whole herd 'underwritten'; with Orbeseal and selected infected cows receive antibiotic DCT as well. Antibiotic DCT is most commonly administered to all quarters of any cows identified as having an infected quarter; however, some producers use antibiotic DCT only on infected quarters, consequently a cow may receive Orbeseal in all four quarters and only antibiotic DCT in, say, one or two (infected) quarters. If more than two quarters are infected, it is advisable to treat all four with antibiotic DCT. CMT is used on individual quarter milk on two occasions in the final week before the expected dry off date to identify infected quarters and therefore infected cows.

- *Pros*: uninfected cows protected and protection of all cows in late dry period.
- *Cons*: as for 3 above, but at least *all* cows are protected, so if cured by antibiotic DCT they will be protected.

5 ALL COWS ORBESEAL ONLY

Limited use, but often favoured by organic herds, but there are potentially serious consequences of escalating BMSCC, particularly if *Staphylococcus aureus* is present in the herd.

6 BLANKET APPROACH – ALL COWS BOTH ORBESEAL AND ANTIBIOTIC DCT

Often used in larger herds where assessment of all cows with CMT before drying off is not practicable, particularly in the light of the limitations of the tools available to determine whether cows are infected or uninfected.

- *Pros*: all cows have opportunity to be cured if they are infected; all cows gain some protection from Orbeseal.
- *Cons*: blanket treatment method, with no diagnosis directing approach; however, in the author's experience, many herds using method 2 (all cows antibiotic DCT

only) see an improvement in udder health when blanket Orbeseal is introduced. This is most likely to be due to the effective 'capture' of cows cured in the dry period, by preventing many from becoming reinfected in the late dry period. The consequence is perhaps at first sight unexpected, as there is often an improvement in the dry-period cure rate as a result of introducing a non-antibiotic preparation.

Herd protocols for the approach to cows due to dry off

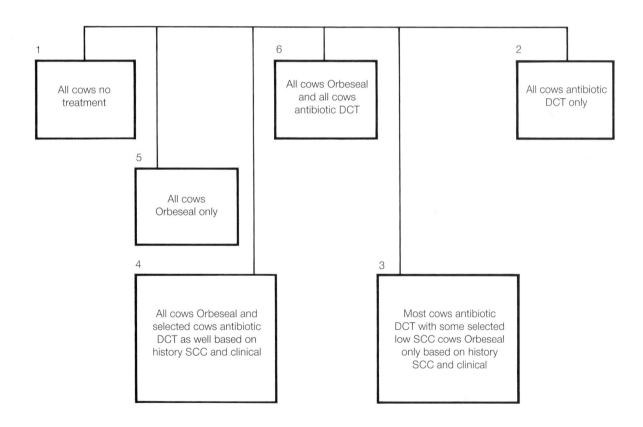

APPENDIX V

Milk Marketing in the United Kingdom

The Milk Marketing Board (MMB) was set up in 1933 to ensure that supplies of affordable milk were available throughout the country. The MMB bought all the milk from the suppliers and sold it on at a standard price to retailers. By 1948 the MMB was collecting milk from 130,000 farmers, using some 500,000 10gall milk churns and delivering to about 10,000 destinations, mainly dairies but also chocolate factories, dried milk factories and other users. Rationalization reduced the number of individual consumer locations supplied to 496 by 1972. Pressure from the MMB, this time on the producer, meant that by the end of the 1970s the once commonplace churns had disappeared, replaced by bulk handling and chilling equipment on the farms in the form of a bulk tank. Refrigerated bulk tanks are still the method for the farm storage of milk awaiting collection, although they are now more technologically advanced and efficient.

This system of milk marketing continued until the MMB was disbanded in 1994. After sixty-one years of board marketing few farmers had any experience of marketing their milk. In 1994 this deregulation of the industry allowed milk to be purchased by many first-time buyers. One consequence of this was an increase in the variability of the price paid to producers. Initially most producers joined the successor to the MMB, a farmer-owned co-operative Milk Marque and accepted lower prices. Milk Marque provided a pool marketing service for its members which predominantly used the same marketing techniques as the MMB had used. Neither the farmers nor industry voted for the deregulation of the milk market. As is often the case, it was the result of the European Union requiring more transparency and a 'level playing field' on price negotiations. However, soon after the market was opened up in November 1994 the dairy processors voiced that they were not happy with Milk Marque's pricing practices and complained at both the UK (Office of Fair Trade) and EU (Competition Commission) level. It was suggested that Milk Marque was using its position in the marketplace in a manner that might disadvantage consumers. In July 1999 the Commission recommended that Milk Marque, despite being reasonably popular and there being similar bodies in other EU countries, be split into three regional pools.

Three co-operative pools were originally regionally structured with Axis in the Midlands, which merged with Scottish Milk and trades as First Milk, and recently became linked to Robert Wiseman Dairies, Milk Link in the South which continues to trade as Milk Link, and Zenith in the north which merged with The Milk Group to become Dairy Farmers of Britain. Milk processing now has many players, with the most significant including Arla Foods UK, Dairy Crest and Robert Wiseman Dairies. Retailers of milk are also numerous but the vast majority is sold through the supermarkets Morrisons, Sainsbury, Somerfield, Tesco and Waitrose.

It seems that subsequent to these changes the power in the milk marketplace, particularly when marketing margins are considered, shifted to the processors and retailers, and all this, despite the assertions to the Commission, with no discernible advantage to consumers. More recently there has been upward pressure on milk price to the producer, with much of the drive coming from a global recognition that food prices need to rise. However, this has been in some ways mitigated or at least complicated at the farm level by the significant and concurrent global rises in fuel, fertilizer and feed costs, especially when wheat prices are taken as a benchmark.

APPENDIX VI

Teat Dips

GENERAL PRINCIPLES

Application of a germicidal solution to dairy cows' teats, most commonly by dipping or spraying, has become an established management procedure to reduce the rate of new intramammary infections in dairy cows. The overall formulation of these products has to balance the positive benefits of germicidal activity with the negative ones on teat condition of the germicidal fraction and the teat-conditioning benefits of the emollient and humectant fractions. It is generally accepted in the dairy industry that the generic term 'teat dip' is used to describe the germicidal solution, irrespective of whether it is applied by dipping or spraying. Application may be immediately before unit attachment (PrMTD) or immediately after unit removal (PMTD). Details of rationale and technique are covered in the relevant sections of Chapter 4. PMTD has been an integral part of mastitis control plans around the world for many decades and was incorporated in the NIRD five-point plan in the 1960s.

PMTD will exert its greatest influence on new infection rates caused by contagious pathogens such as *Staphylococcus aureus*, *Streptococcus agalactiae* and *Corynebacterium bovis*. PMTD gives little control over contamination that occurs between milkings as the duration of activity falls significantly only a few hours after application. PrMTD, despite being a more recent development, has become increasingly adopted in recent decades. PrMTD will exert its influence by minimizing the number of potential mastitis pathogens on the teat ends prior to unit attachment, thus helping to reduce new infection rates caused by these pathogens, and most notably environmental bacteria such

as *Streptococcus uberis*, *Escherichia coli*, and *Klebsiella pneumoniae*.

The establishment of an intramammary infection generally requires a mastitis-causing pathogen to penetrate through the streak canal and research shows that the incidence and type of mastitis that develops is directly related to the number and types of bacteria on teat skin. Teat disinfection is simple, effective and an economic way to reduce bacterial populations on teat skin, both before and after milking and will help to reduce new intramammary infection rates. However, it must be remembered that there is no effect on existing infections and consequently no rapid reduction in mastitis rates are observed if teat dipping is introduced or effectiveness improved, which is contrary to what the milker is expecting or hoping for.

GENERAL SELECTION OF TEAT DIP TYPE

The aims of PrMTD and PMTD are somewhat different in terms of the speed of onset of action and its duration. There may also be more of a requirement for PMTD to contain significant levels of teat conditioner. This, in the author's opinion, makes dual purpose pre-post dips a compromise in function for both PrMTD and PMTD. The requirements of a disinfectant for use in PrMTD are rapid kill, since contact time will be short. The requirements of a disinfectant for use in PMTD are to try to maintain disinfectant activity for as long as possible, as well as help to maintain teat skin condition. In general, post-milking disinfectants contain more emollients or humectants, such as lanolin, glycerine or sorbitol, and, in an ideal world, a post-milking teat disinfectant would span the time between milkings, thus affording some long-term protection; however, this is not achievable and nor might it be desirable as there would be potential residue issues when the cows were next milked. The compromise between speed and duration of activity is avoidable when choosing teat dips by using different product with different speed of onset and durations of activity for pre- and post-milking disinfection.

HOW THEY ARE APPLIED?

The application of germicidal teat disinfectants is generally done either by dip (including liquid, gel or foaming products) or spray. Details are covered in the relevant sections on PrMTD and PMTD under milking routine in Chapter 4.

HOW ARE THEY STORED AND HANDLED?

Dip chemicals should be stored in such a way as to avoid extremes of temperature. Freezing may cause the separation of product components, while overheating can cause volatilization of product ingredients, with a resulting reduction in germicidal activity and possible pH changes which may cause irritation to teat skin.

All germicidal products are adversely affected by organic matter such as milk, soil or dung. If teat dipping cups become contaminated during milking they should be emptied washed and refilled with fresh dip. Teat dip delivered by spray is not prone to contamination in this way.

CHEMICALS USED AS TEAT DISINFECTANTS WITH TEAT-CONDITIONING PROPERTIES

A variety of germicidal chemicals are suitable for use in food production, with some being commonly included in teat dips, often combined with teat conditioners while others are more frequently found in teat-sanitizing products which will be used more for cleaning equipment or washing teats. Germicidal chemicals used in the dairy environment will include iodine, chlorhexidine, dodecyl benzene sulphonic acid, sodium hypochlorite, quaternary ammonium, chlorine-based products such as acidified sodium chlorite and hydrogen peroxide-based products. These chemicals destroy bacteria by a variety of mechanisms, including chemical or biological action such as oxidation-reduction, denaturation/precipitation of cytoplasmic proteins, inhibition of enzyme activity and disruption of cell membranes.

GERMICIDAL CHEMICAL GROUPS USED IN TEAT DIPS

Iodophor-based Dips

These are the most commonly used and have a variety of manufacturers. Iodine is a fast-acting, broad-spectrum germicide which is effective against most mastitis-causing bacteria, fungi, bacterial spores and some viruses as a result of an oxidizing reaction between iodine and organic matter. Iodophor teat dips enable most of the iodine to be present in a bound and inactive form by creating a complex with water-soluble detergents or surfactants. It is the free iodine as the uncomplexed form (usually 6 to 12ppm) that provides the antimicrobial activity by oxidizing microorganisms. There is a chemical equilibrium between the free (active) and the complexed (inactive) iodine so that as the free iodine is used up as it comes into contact with organic matter it is immediately replaced from the complexed iodine. Thus free iodine is always available, maintaining a germicidal effect until the total amount of available iodine in the iodophor has been depleted.

The need to use detergents as complexing agents in iodophor teat dips tends to result in the removal of natural protective oils from the teat skin, requiring the addition of teat conditioners. Common conditioners include moisturizers such as glycerine or propylene at between 2 and 10 per cent, sometimes combined with lanolin as an emollient to replace natural oils lost from the skin. Iodophors are perhaps the most commonly used teat dips and are available as both pre- and post-conventional dips and barrier type products. The characteristic brown coloration helps to identify the coverage of the teat (or lack of coverage) once applied which contributes to their popularity.

Chlorine-based Dips

The halogens are rapidly acting, destroying a wide range of microbes. Chlorine is commonly used as a disinfectant in a variety of forms. Generally, the activity of made-up, chlorine-based teat dips declines over time as they have a short shelf life and must be used within hours of preparation. There are two commonly used types of chlorine product described below.

Acidified Sodium Chlorite

Acidified sodium chlorite products, such as Udder Gold, combine sodium chlorite with an appropriate acid or acids, such as lactic acid or mandelic acid, resulting in the active components, chlorous acid and chlorine dioxide. These have a broad spectrum of action against mastitis-causing bacteria as well as moulds, yeasts and viruses and they generally include teat-conditioning humectants and emollients. They are available as two-part systems made up of equal volumes of an activator and a base, which must be mixed and prepared daily to provide optimal antimicrobial activity. Some products have a gel formulation, which forms a protective barrier over the teat end and may prolong the killing action of the chlorous acid.

Chlorhexidine

Chlorhexidine is a rapidly acting, generally non-irritant disinfectant. It is active against most bacteria and some molds, yeasts and viruses by action on the cell wall. It is bacteriostatic at low concentrations and bactericidal at higher concentrations, with the levels depending on the bacteria. If the dip is heavily contaminated,

for example in a dip cup, *Serratia* species and *Pseudomonas* species can survive and serve as potential mastitis pathogens.

Chlorhexidine is commonly used at 0.5 per cent in teat products. It adheres well to teat skin, provides some prolonged activity and products generally contain humectants and emollients to minimize irritation, although it does not have a significantly deleterious effect on teat skin. Both conventional and barrier teat formulations are available. Hibiscrub is often used by both veterinary and medical surgeons for the preparation of hands and the surgical site before surgery.

Dodecyl Benzene Sulphonic Acid (DDBSA)

Teat dip products containing DDBSA, such as Blu Gard, are generally non-irritant but often have teat-conditioning products such as glycerine added, as well as organic acids to maintain the pH around 3.0 for maximum efficacy. They are effective against most mastitis-causing bacteria as well as yeasts and are available as conventional or barrier formulations.

Quaternary Ammonium

This disinfectant is generally used at 0.05 to 1.0 per cent and causes little skin irritation, provided that the pH is balanced and teat skin conditioners are added. High levels of organic contamination will reduce efficacy and, as with chlorhexidine disinfectant, *Serratia* species and *Pseudomonas* species have been known to survive in quaternary ammonium teat dips.

Sodium Hypochlorite

Sodium hypochlorite solutions are more commonly known as household bleach. Although such solutions are not marketed as teat dips, they continue to be used by some farmers as both pre- and post-milking dips. Dilution is necessary to avoid damage to teat skin and the final concentration of sodium hydroxide must be less than 0.5 per cent. Emollients cannot be included because of adverse interactions. Hypochlorite is a strong oxidizing agent and is active against most bacteria, viruses and molds. However, it is an irritant and may cause some inflammation to both the teats and milkers' hands if gloves are not worn. Often this is transient and after a period of 'getting used to it' the teat condition will improve. Hypochlorite is best seen as a dairy disinfectant rather than a teat dip and its use cannot be recommended.

Hydrogen Peroxide

This disinfectant (for instance, Sorgene) provides a wide spectrum of control against most mastitis-causing bacteria through its strong oxidizing action. Generally used as a dairy disinfectant, it will cause teat irritation, much like hypochlorite. Most commonly used for cluster disinfection between cows at a dilution of between 500:1 (0.2 per cent) with 50ml of peracetic acid in a 25ltr drum of water, up to a dilution of 200:1 (0.5 per cent), with 125ml in a 25ltr drum of water. Often farms use something in between, such as using 80ml in a 25ltr drum of water, resulting in just over 0.3 per cent solution.

APPENDIX VII: Interpretation of the Significance of Isolates from Milk Sample Types

Sample type	Bacteria isolated	Comment
Clinical sample Milk generally visually abnormal Would include repeat cases	**Any** bacteria (pathogen)	in pure and profuse growth is likely to be significant; will include potential contaminants such as *Streptococcus faecalis* or *Protatheca* In author's opinion mixed infections do occur, e.g. *Streptococcus uberis* and *E.coli*, but when multiple pathogens are isolated from a clinical sample interpretation is more difficult, – particularly if cfus are low; contamination cannot be ruled out 'No growth' is a special case in clinical cases – *E.coli* may not be viable in the udder or the milk sample for more than a few hours and consequently a proportion of no growths may well be environmental mastitis cases; use clinical judgement to help interpretation
High SCC sample Milk generally visually normal Also include post-treatment checks	**Major pathogens**	In author's view, always significant even if mixed with contaminant pathogens;
	Staphylococcus aureus *Streptococcus agalactiae*	As minimum, demonstrates that they exist in the herd. Repeat sampling of HSCC cows will indicate importance to herd economics and health
	Minor pathogens	Possible normal commensal organisms – possible protective role of minor pathogens? can be significant in their own right – depends on cfus and other pathogens isolated – can originate from teat surface
	Coag –ve Staphylococcus	Many cows calve with *Coag –ve Staphylococcus* but self-cure; see text on coagulase test
	Coryne bovis	May indicate poor post-milking teat disinfection; can give rise to elevated BMSCCs if high enough prevalence
	Other pathogens	Other pathogens can give rise to persistent infections and so result in prolonged elevation of SCCs; again depends on cfus and other pathogens isolated
	Streptococcus uberis	Genetic fingerprinting has demonstrated persistent infection with associated elevation of SCC. very likely to be significant if pure and profuse growth isolated from high SCC quarters May have a contagious component in spread; of major concern in author's practice
	Strep dysgalactiae	Generally responds well to treatment – author's view unlikely to result in herd BMSCC rises Associated with poor teat condition and blackspot – problems with teat condition may give relatively high prevalence
	Coliform – E.coli *Strep faecalis*	In author's view unlikely to give rise to significant numbers of persistent infections which result in elevation of SCC and in turn elevation of BMSCC; generally put down as contamination in HSCC samples However, repeat isolation of pure and significant cfus would indicate persistent infection
	Non-specific pathogens	An open mind; with repeat culture of pathogens not expected to give rise to persistent infections and elevation of SCCs will allow for the unusual sub-clinical cases; *see text on Protatheca*
	No growth	Again a special case. This could indicate no significant bacteria are present. The cell count rise could be due to severe damage to the udder and, in fact, a bacteriological cure has been achieved or intermittent excretion, with say *Staphylococcus aureus*, has meant that there were insufficient bacteria to culture on the day of sampling; *see intermittent serial quarter testing (ISQT) to improve chances of isolating Staphylococcus aureus*

APPENDIX VIII

Specific Treatment Protocols

INTRODUCTION

Insufficient data exist to differentiate the efficacy of different antimicrobials for different types of intrammamry infection, let alone for different treatment protocols or different manifestations of those infections. It is not the purpose here to indicate or direct the reader to certain treatment protocols. However, this section lists a few treatment approaches that the author has found to be useful in certain circumstances.

It must be remembered that, while specific treatment protocols used on cows selected for their increased likelihood of cure may help to reduce the duration of infections in those cows treated (which may in turn reduce the likely spread of bacteria within a herd) the importance of the control of intramammary infections by management protocols, such as ensuring a clean, dry cow environment and a sound hygienic milking routine, remains.

Treatment protocols will involve drug regimens which are not as found in the Marketing Authority (drug licence) for those products and, as such, will be 'off label' use. There are important considerations when using drugs in ways other than those described on the label. It is only when they are used according to the manufacturer's label that they are granted a licence to be used in food-producing animals. The granting of a licence in the United Kingdom requires considerable data on safety, efficacy and environmental considerations, and when the drug is used in the way described on the label it will have specific milk and meat withhold periods. Any deviation in the recommended number of treatments, frequency, dose or duration of treatment will void that licensed milk and a meat withhold and trigger a minimum 'standard' milk withhold of seven days and a meat withhold of twenty-eight.

For the above reasons 'off-label treatment' should:

*   only be undertaken only under the supervision of the veterinary surgeon who has the animals under his or her care;
*   include a written SOP to be given to the farmer (with a copy being retained by the practice), detailing the drugs to be used and routes of administration, with doses and timing. The SOP should also state that there is a minimum seven-day milk withhold and twenty-eight-day meat withhold, and suggest that the milk is tested with Delvo SP before it is returned to the tank; the form should also record the date of treatment and the farmer's name and address, along with the cow's identity and the quarter(s) treated. The author has individual SOPs for the off-label treatment protocols used in his veterinary practice;
*   be directed at cows where there is sufficient information to justify off-label treatment in terms of improved cure rates and reduced recurrence rates.

Research shows that, particularly with Gram-positive infections such as *Staphylococcus aureus* or some strains of *Streptococcus uberis*, increasing duration, frequency and, on occasions, varying the route of administration can significantly increase the chance of successful treatment. Work also shows that, when looked at over a longer period of time overall, the total drug usage can be reduced, despite the increased dose or duration of drugs used on an individual case. This is because the 'true' treatment success in terms of bacteriological cure and the elimination of the causative bacteria is improved, resulting in fewer recurrent cases from infections, which, with less intense treatment, are often clinically cured but remain infected, only to recur at some later date.

Treatments listed here are generally used after a laboratory diagnosis and the causal pathogen has been identified. In some circumstances a herd may be having on-going problems with a specific pathogen and not all cases will justify sampling. Product withholds where stated assume twice daily milking.

STAPHYLOCOCCUS AUREUS

During Lactation

On-label
Often the chance of successful treatment during lactation is small and, although many and varied off-label protocols exist, the author tends to use a label course of Orbenin LA. In his opinion, the strain of *Staphylococcus aureus* and the duration of infection are greater influences on the treatment outcome than the treatment used. Although success rates in lactation are poor if culling is not possible of all *Staphylococcus aureus*-infected cows (a common situation) then suppression of excretion, albeit temporarily, is a useful outcome of therapy in the battle to reduce spread within the herd. As long as everyone knows bacteriological cure is unlikely and that the cows will probably be culled eventually, this in the author's opinion is still acceptable.

- Cloxacillin 200mg (Orbenin LA, Pfizer Animal Health) – label treatment; three tubes at 48hr intervals with an 84hr milk withhold (milk taken from seventh milking).

At Drying Off or Before Calving

Off-label
This requires a minimum seven-day milk and twenty-eight-day meat withhold – and test milk. Herds known to have *Staphylococcus aureus*-infected cows should use antibiotic dry cow on all cows at drying off. The author favours long-acting Cloxacillin-based preparations in this situation. Additional treatment can be useful at drying off and, in his experience, the use of:

- Tilmicosin 300mg (Micotil Elanco Animal Health) at drying off: 1ml per 30kg administered in divided doses at multiple sites under the skin at drying off give the best results. The author uses 20ml for a 600kg cow, administering 5ml at four different sites. However, case selection (choosing cows likely to get better) influences the success rate greatly. Cows with recent infections (identified either by individual SCC, if available, or by lactational age, if not) are more likely to respond. Micotil *must* be administered by a veterinary surgeon.
- Tylosin 200mg/ml (Tylan Elanco Animal Health): 100ml given under the skin in two divided doses, either at drying off or pre-calving as the cow starts to spring to calve and the udder starts to develop (seven to ten days before calving) can also improve cure rates.

As both Tilmicosin and Tylosin are 'acid trapped' or 'pH trapped' there are some benefits in treating a few days before drying off. These drugs are attracted to acid conditions in the body and often even the infected lactating gland has a lower pH than a dry udder (an infected lung is also slightly acidic), which is why these drugs concentrate in the udder and lung. However, there are dangers that, if several people are responsible for milking the herd, the milk from a treated cow which is close to drying off may be inadvertently included in the bulk milk tank, causing an antibiotic violation. Continuing to milk the cow after administration confers a theoretical advantage that the drug is drawn into the udder in higher concentrations, but this must be weighed against the risk of a significant financial penalty if antibiotics are detected in the farm bulk milk tank.

STREPTOCOCCUS UBERIS

During Lactation
Streptococcus uberis is perhaps not as commonly recognized as a persistent infection within the

mammary gland, but research performed in the author's practice in collaboration with Dr Maureen Milne of Glasgow University and other research workers has shown that *Streptococcus uberis* infection can indeed be resilient to label treatment. The author tends to favour extended aggressive treatment in selected cows. But those with long histories of high SCC or clinical cases over several lactations are unlikely to respond and may justify culling.

Off-label

This requires a minimum seven-day milk and twenty-eight-day meat withhold – and test milk.

The author's approach is either:

- Six tubes of either Cefquinome 75mg (Cobactan LC, Intervet, United Kingdom) or penethamate hydriodide 150mg, dihydrostreptomycin 150mg, Framycetin sulphate 50 mg, Prednisolone 5mg (Ubro Yellow, Boehringer Ingelheim Ltd at 12hr intervals (every milking), concurrently with four days of penethamate hydriodide (Mamyzin, Boehringer Ingelheim Ltd) (10g on day one and 5g daily for the next three days), or
- Six tubes of either Cobactan LC or Ubro Yellow at 12hr intervals (every milking), concurrently with four days of Tylosin 200mg/ml (Tylan, Elanco Animal Health) (20ml at 12hr intervals on three occasions then 20ml once daily on two occasions).

At Drying Off or before Calving

The author's opinion is that, since the advent of a blanket herd approach of the concurrent use of internal teat seal (Orbeseal) and antibiotic dry cow therapy at drying off, additional parentral antibiotic treatment at drying off or pre-calving is perhaps less critical for known *Streptococcus uberis*-infected cows at drying off. The treatment at drying off may well have cured an intramammary infection only for the cow to pick up another infection just before calving. A pre-calving treatment protocol helps to reduce this, but would allow existing infections to persist longer before

they were treated. If cure rates with antibiotic DCT are reasonable for many cows infected with *Streptococcus uberis* at drying off, then the internal teat seal may well protect these cows from reinfection.

However, if dry cow performance indicates poor cure rates then selected cows may justify treatment at or before calving as discussed earlier under *Staphylococcus aureus*. For *Streptococcus uberis the* author tends to use Tylosin 200mg/ml (Tylan, Elanco Animal Health).

Heifers Pre-calving

Heifers do not generally have the advantage of either an internal teat seal or antibiotic DCT to protect or eliminate any infections acquired before they calve. It is well recognized that heifers calving in can be just as prone to acquire new infections in the days running up to calving as cows are. As a result, groups of dairy heifers have, on occasions, had both or either antibiotic DCT and/or teat seal (Orbeseal, Pfizer Animal Health) administered a few weeks prior to the expected calving date in an attempt to reduce intramammary infection rates, although the author has no experience of this and would not recommend it. In particularly hot summers the author has experienced heifers 'camping' under trees for shade and acquiring infection from faecal contamination in and around the area. This has led to an increase in the number of heifers calving in with *Streptococcus uberis* infections in many herds. Work from around the world, including the United Kingdom, has shown a reduction in the number of heifers calving with *Streptococcus uberis* infection that have received penethamate hydriodide (Mamyzin, Boehringer Ingelheim Ltd) at or around calving. The author is currently (2008) involved in a trial where heifers receive 10g Mamyzin on the day of calving and again 24hr later. The pre-calving use of any injectable antibiotic, while perhaps more logical in this situation, is not easy in heifers, as it is notoriously difficult to predict when a heifer is going to calve. If the heifer does not calve within a few days of the treatment it would need to be repeated, adding to cost and the unnecessary use of antibiotic.

Inhibitory Substance Tests

Inhibitory substances found in milk collected from a bulk milk tank are rare but would most likely be as a result of human error in allowing a cow's milk with antibiotic residues, either under treatment or within the milk withhold period into the bulk tank. However, it is worth bearing in mind that cows can produce naturally occurring inhibitory substances and that the contamination of milk by disinfectants would, in theory, result in the failure of an inhibitory substance test, although this would be more likely to be at the individual cow level. Milk for human consumption can be screened by a variety of tests, including non-specific inhibitory substance tests and more specific antibiotic tests. Some screening tests work by detecting an inhibitory substance that prevents a very sensitive bacterium (*Bacillus stearothermophilus*) to grow. When the sample is incubated, the growth of the bacteria changes the pH of the test medium, causing an indicator dye to change colour from purple to yellow. If antibiotics (or other inhibitory substances) are present in the milk being tested, this inhibits the growth of the bacteria, prevents the pH change, no colour change occurs and the test medium remains purple.

Research has shown that this test, originally developed for churn milk testing, has some limitations when testing an individual cow's milk. Despite this, DelvoSP is probably the most commonly used cow-side test by farmers. Freshly calved cows, especially if they have a high SCC, can produce enough natural inhibitory substances to fail the test. The DelvoSP is unlikely to be affected by natural inhibitory substances, except when single cows are being tested, in which case it is reasonable to dilute the milk from a freshly calved cow that calves early (within the minimum dry period of the DCT used) to check for antibiotic with, say, five bulk tank milk to one test cow milk.

From a consumer safety point of view, the test is more likely to give a false positive than a false negative result, thus protecting the supply chain. This false positive would also apply if the test were not incubated at the correct temperature.

There is also a theoretical possibility that DelvoSP can detect some antibiotics (mainly the semi-synthetic penicillins) below the maximum residue limit (MRL), the amount set in Europe for each and every antibiotic permitted to be used in food-producing animals, and what the withdrawal periods are, not surprisingly, based on. It is therefore, in theory, possible for milk to be technically and legally fit for human consumption (below the MRL for all antibiotics) but fail the DelvoSP test. Experience from the processing dairies suggests that most antibiotic failures at a farm level are such that the levels are many times higher than the MRL, and when bulk milk is tested the theoretical possibility of the DelvoSP test giving an incorrect positive (that is, despite being below the MRL) is so small as to be ignored. Nonetheless, this could set a precedent and, as technology advances and test sensitivity increases, we could find milk buyers demanding levels considerably below the MRL just because they can. This would not seem logical nor fair as the MRL is set in Europe by food safety experts and has a significant safety margin built in.

More specific tests such as ßeta s.t.a.r. are now used in many UK processing dairies, and to a lesser extent CHARM and SNAP, to screen milk. These detect the presence of the beta lactam ring, a chemical structure found in all penicillin-based intramammary treatments, including penicillin, semi-synthetic penicillins such as Ampicillin, Amoxicillin and the cephalosporins. A positive result to this test is specific and indicates the presence of a beta lactam antibiotic.

Further Reading

BOOKS AND CONFERENCE PROCEEDINGS

Proceedings, 1980 BCVA, *Mastitis Control and Herd Management*, Technical Bulletin (4) (NIRD, Hannah Research Institute), ed. Bramley, Dodd and Griffin, ISBN 0 7084 0195 3

Bramley, Dodd and Jackson (eds), *Control of Bovine Mastitis*, BCVA, 1971.

Bramley, Dodd and Mein (eds), *Machine Milking and Lactation*, Insight Books, 1992, ISBN 0 9519188 0 X.

Blowey and Edmondson, *Mastitis Control in Dairy Herds*, Farming Press, 1995, ISBN 0 85236 314 1.

Proceedings, IDF Conferences, Tel Aviv, 1995 and Maastricht, 2005.

USEFUL WEBSITES

BMC: proceedings of conferences, 1998: www.iah.bbsrc.ac.uk/bmc/index.html

BCVA: proceedings, 1993– with membership: www.bcva.org.uk/

NMC: proceedings, factsheets, resources, some without membership: www.nmconline.org/

AABP: proceedings, factsheets, resources, some without membership: www.aabp.org/

IDF: www.fil-idf.org/Content/Default.asp

IAH: www.iah.ac.uk/

UKVet: www.ukvet.co.uk/

NOAH: www.noah.co.uk/

Dutch Udder Health Centre: www.ugcn.nl/

Canadian Bovine Mastitis Research Network: www.medvet.umontreal.ca/reseau_mammite/producteurs/index.php?page=accueil

Milk Recording Companies

NMR: www.nmr.co.uk/

CIS: www.thecis.co.uk/

Dairy Industry Websites

DeLaval: www.delaval.com/default.htm

ADF: www.ad-f.com/Eng/home.htm

Cluster Flush: www.vaccar.com/; www.cluster-flush.com/index.html

Assured Dairy Farms (ADF – formerly NDFAS): www.ndfas.org.uk/

DairyCo (formerly MDC): www.mdc.org.uk/

MDC Datum: www.mdcdatum.org.uk/

MDC Datum Milk Quality: www.mdcdatum.org.uk/MilkSupply/milkquality.html

Spreadsheet Calculators

The following simple spreadsheet calculators are available from the author at ValeLab@btinternet.com

- *Liner Replacement Calculator*: input the number of cows milked, frequency of milking and milking units, and the liner replacement interval is displayed as both an interval in days/months and a frequency as the number of times a year

- *Hidden Quarter*: two-part calculator, enter uninfected and infected quarter SCC and the cow SCC will display; enter uninfected quarters and a cow SCC and the worst quarter SCC will display; uninfected quarters are assumed to have the same SCC and all four quarters the same yield.

Index

Index